Anti-Inflammatory Keto (30% More Effective)

Complete Beginners Guide to the Ketogenic Low-Carb Clarity with Intermittent Fasting for Accelerated Results; Reset your Life Today and Slim Down Forever

Christine Moore

© Copyright 2019 - All rights reserved.

The content contained within this book may not be reproduced, duplicated or transmitted without direct written permission from the author or the publisher.

Under no circumstances will any blame or legal responsibility be held against the publisher, or author, for any damages, reparation, or monetary loss due to the information contained within this book. Either directly or indirectly.

Legal Notice:
This book is copyright protected. This book is only for personal use. You cannot amend, distribute, sell, use, quote or paraphrase any part, or the content within this book, without the consent of the author or publisher.

Disclaimer Notice:

Please note the information contained within this document is for educational and entertainment purposes only. All effort has been executed to present accurate, up to date, and reliable, complete information. No warranties of any kind are declared or implied. Readers acknowledge that the author is not engaging in the rendering of legal, financial, medical or professional advice. The content within this book has been derived from various sources. Please consult a licensed professional before attempting any techniques outlined in this book.

By reading this document, the reader agrees that under no circumstances is the author responsible for any losses, direct or indirect, which are incurred as a result of the use of information contained within this document, including, but not limited to, — errors, omissions, or inaccuracies.

Contents

Introduction _____ 1

Chapter 1:
The Ketogenic Diet _____ 4

Chapter 2:
Ketosis _____ 11

Chapter 3:
The Nutritional Break Down _____ 19

Chapter 4:
Dirty Keto _____ 23

Chapter 5:
The Mediterranean Diet _____ 31

Chapter 6:
Ketogenic Mediterranean Diet _____ 42

Chapter 7:
Keto-Mediterranean Vegetables _____ 51

Chapter 8:
Keto Mediterranean Meats and Nuts _____ 56

Chapter 9:
Keto-Mediterranean Fruits and Dairy Products _____ 67

Chapter 10:
Finding Your Carb Sweet Spot _____ 76

Chapter 11:
Intermittent Fasting _____ 90

Chapter 12:
The Mediterranean Ketogenic Diet _____ 100

Chapter 13:
Foods to Eat on IF and Sample Meal Plan _____ 104

Chapter 14:
Fourteen: Common Mistakes _____ 110

Chapter 15:
Tips and Tricks _____ 116

Chapter 16:
Frequently Asked Questions _____ 128

Conclusion _____ 141

CHRISTINE MOORE

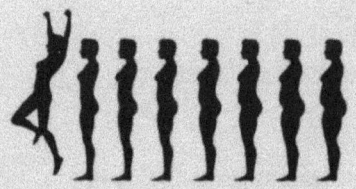

ANTI-INFLAMMATORY
KETO
30 PERCENT
MORE *Effective*

COMPLETE WOMEN AND MEN BEGINNERS GUIDE TO THE
KETOGENIC LOW-CARB CLARITY WITH INTERMITTENT FASTING
FOR ACCELERATED WEIGHT LOSS; RESET YOUR LIFE TODAY

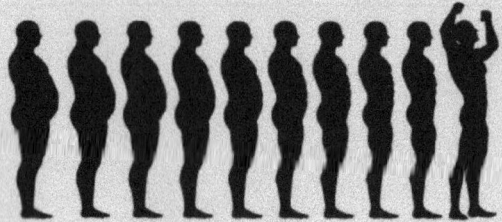

Introduction

If you are looking for a way to get healthier and eat better, then this is the right book for you. Health should always be one of our foremost concerns, with diet being one of the main factors that affect our health. Due to the booming food industry and consumerism, among other factors, our diets have undergone a very drastic and unhealthy change.

Our dietary choices are often influenced by advertisements and packaging that aim to financially benefit food corporations rather than human health. The widely available and extremely cheap junk food and processed food options found in supermarket shelves have directly contributed to unhealthy food choices and increased weight issues.

If you compare statistics from your grandparent's times to recent years, you will notice the increase in obesity, type 2 diabetes, eating disorders, among other health concerns. As a result of these issues, there is higher concern with healthy weight loss and dieting, but often people get caught up on fad diets that are not necessarily effective. The purpose of this book is to present information about the Keto-

Mediterranean diet and the many benefits associated with each diet individually, as well as the diets in combination with one another.

You may have heard of the Ketogenic and Mediterranean diets, even if you're not very familiar with the specifics of each. In this book, the details of each will be discussed, alongside, how they can improve your personal well-being and ways in which you can implement them.

These days' people have become more conscious of the ingredients that go in the preparation of their food. There is more awareness about all the harmful additives and preservatives in processed food. For this reason, the focus is shifting to eating more wholesome and natural food.

Through learning about the ketogenic diet, you will also learn how our ancestors ate and why following such a diet is still beneficial for our health today. Illness and weight issues were relatively non-existent in older times compared to now. Furthermore, the Mediterranean diet is a heart-friendly diet. These are not fad diets, and we have considered various factors before recommending them for the benefit of the reader. You don't have to stop eating everything you like or sit and count the ingredients in all you ate. You don't have to switch to a liquid diet or eat only once a day.

For many years, fat was considered the culprit behind increased weight concerns, but it is not true at all. Fat is an important part of your diet. So, stop listening to all the false information that you may be bombarded with. Instead, we will explain everything about the foods that will benefit your health and how you can switch to a healthy and still appealing diet.

It is very important to make conscious decisions about what you pick up at the store or and cook with. Good food choices will not only have a very significant impact on weight loss and management, but also improving overall physical and mental health. As you read on, you will learn how you can do this with the help of the Ketogenic Mediterranean diet. You will be able to eat good wholesome and delicious food that will benefit your health for years to come.

Chapter 1:
The Ketogenic Diet

This chapter will introduce the fundamentals of the Ketogenic (Keto) diet, how it works, and transitioning your body from running on carbohydrates (i.e. carbs) to running on fats. The ketogenic diet should be thought of more as a lifestyle; it doesn't set unrealistic and unhealthy rules about what you should or should not eat, or how much and how often. You won't have to curb your hunger with only boiled vegetables, or switch to raw shakes instead of wholesome meals.

The ketogenic lifestyle is not a demanding fad diet that will require immense self-control and stress you out about your food and weight. You won't have to starve yourself at any point either. This diet helps you understand what is good for your body and what is detrimental towards your health. You will automatically choose to make choices that will benefit you and not harm you.

The food corporations usually lie about the nutritious value about the foods they are trying to sell and make you believe that food labeled low fat or fat-free is healthy for you. All this is just a sham to mislead you and make you purchase their products. Recently, scientists and nutritionists have started endorsing the fact that our ancestors were much healthier than us and this was due to their healthier diets. The ketogenic diet recommends that we all shift back to that healthy diet again. There is a reason your grandma complains about what you constantly snack on. The older generations ate much more wholesome foods and thus managed to stay fit and healthy.

Our processed diets are doing nothing to benefit us. You must realize that everything you are told is not true, especially when it comes to the negative stigma that has become attached to fats. Most people in recent years have blamed fats as the main culprit behind any issues related to foods. But there are healthy fats that are essential for good health. Therefore, you should not follow any diets that eliminate fat from your food. Basing your food choices on correct facts or information is important.

If your main concern is excess weight, you need to understand the reason why you gained it in the first place. It is not always due to excessive eating but more about what you are eating. As mentioned already, it is not all due to fat either. The real culprit is the processed food that the food industry pushes for their profit and at the cost of our good health. The fat that occurs naturally in meat, dairy and other natural sources is good for health. The corporations are who have pushed the blame for bad health on fat for their benefit over the past couple of decades.

With the growing processed food industry, you will notice the rise in food-related issues as well. Type 2 Diabetes is one of the diseases that increased alarmingly with this. This was not the case even a few decades ago. You can see that fats are not the blame and instead you should eliminate unhealthy processed food from your diet. Another evil in your diet is sugar that must be removed or controlled. This ingredient causes only harm and has no nutritional benefit whatsoever for your health. Sugar and not fats can cause an alarming increase in your body weight too. You probably don't even realize how much-refined sugar is present in most of the processed food you consume. You can see how the industry has gained enough power to control our eating habits for their gain. When people notice that they gain weight, they start eating less or following fad diets. Instead of doing that, you can try to opt for healthier diet options like the ketogenic diet.

The ketogenic diet tells you to eat more like our ancestors, but with a decrease in the number of carbohydrates consumed while increasing the quantity of fats, thus pushing the body to burn fat as fuel. The purpose behind this strategy is to keep the body in a constant state of ketosis because, instead of banning fats from your diet, you will benefit more by majorly reducing your carbohydrate consumptions.

The demonization of fats is not going to help you in any way. Refined carbohydrates are more detrimental to your health and need to be reduced especially if you want to lose weight. Don't follow fad diets that leave you hungry for hours at a time. At some point, you will have to give in to hunger and then end up binge eating, fats help you feel full longer, preventing food cravings that can contribute to excess eating. You can eat all your regular meals with a heightened level of consciousness about the ingredients that you consume. The Keto also advocates for moderate consumption of proteins, which can also be obtained from wholesome and nutritious sources. There are many reports of people who have tried the keto diet found it to be helpful in losing weight, increasing stamina, and observing overall health improvements.

The ketogenic diet's name refers to the ketones and ketosis that occur in the human body as a result of the food that is consumed and used as the main source of energy. A constantly induced state of ketosis will help the body utilize stored fat for fuel; this includes excess fat stored in the liver, helping to reduce the likelihood of Fatty Liver Disease. The main thing that you learn from the ketogenic diet is that fats are not what cause obesity, heart attacks and all the other problems that they are usually blamed for. So, start adding them back into your diet liberally, if the fats that you decide to eat are from the right sources. You might be skeptical about this but take a chance, and you will not regret it.

Benefits of The Ketogenic Diet

Reducing carbohydrates will reduce excess triglycerides in the body. The keto diet helps in blood pressure regulation and will prevent heart issues and hardening of arteries as well.

High levels of insulin in the body can cause polycystic ovary syndrome in women. The ketogenic diet helps to reduce this excess insulin in the body and thus lowers risk of PCOD, which can be harmful to women and causes problems in conception and fertility.

You will also see that there is less occurrence of acid reflux or heartburn since these are increased by consumption of carbs like potatoes or foods containing sugars.

Certain studies show that the ketogenic diet benefits patients who have epilepsy and cancer; however, this is still being researched on, and no concrete evidence supports it.

Due to the benefits that the keto diet has on brain health, it can also reduce the risk of conditions like Alzheimer's or Parkinson's disease.

Another benefit is that the keto diet keeps a healthy check on uric acid levels in the body. If it is too much, it can cause gout or kidney stone formation, but the keto diet regulates it.

It is evident that there are a lot of benefits associated with following the ketogenic diet. For this reason, we recommend that you try the Keto diet for yourself.

Anti-Inflammatory Keto (30% More Effective)

Precautions

Before you follow any specific diet, you should consult a doctor. They will help you in deciding which diet is the most appropriate for your body and if there are any that might have a detrimental effect on your health. Every person's body is different and has its own needs. You cannot expect the same diet to work for every person and to have the same results. There are certain health issues or conditions as well that might make a certain diet or certain ingredients unsuitable for your body. Consultation from a doctor will help you to avoid any unwanted health issue aggravations. They will instead guide you so that you can reap the maximum benefit from the diet in a healthy way.

Note that those who have diseases related to the liver, kidney or pancreas should avoid the keto diet. The diet is also not suited for anyone who has muscular dystrophy. It is helpful for patients of diabetes type two and should not be followed by patients who have diabetes type one. Gestational diabetes does not react well with the ketogenic diet in the body.

Pregnant and nursing women have different nutritional requirements and should always consult their doctors as changing diets may affect their and their infant's health. Someone who suffers from eating disorders should always consult a doctor before following any specific diet. Their focus should be on regaining health, and the doctor will determine if the ketogenic diet is appropriate for such patients. Strict diets can often backfire for people with eating disorders when they should be focusing on healthier eating. These are just some precautions that we recommend you keep in mind before you start following the ketogenic diet or any such diet blindly. This diet is a safe and healthy diet that a lot of people have tried and benefited from; however, certain illnesses or conditions of the body require special care that you need to make sure you provide to stay healthy.

Side Effects of The Ketogenic Diet

As with any change in behavior, there may be some side effects when you initially start the keto diet. These side effects are usually temporary and pass over time and with care. Pay extra attention if you suffer from any medical conditions or take medications that might react adversely with the ketogenic diet.

One of the most common side effects is hypoglycemia, which causes dizziness, fatigue and irritability. This will pass after a few weeks, but to address it effectively, frequently eat small meals and stay hydrated throughout the day. Also, consider adding or maintaining enough sodium into your diet.

Other side effects can be caused by HPA axis dysfunction, which refers to the three glands; hypothalamus, pituitary and adrenal. You can deal with the associated condition with the help of apoptogenic herbs, blood sugar regulation and hydration.

Chapter 2:
Ketosis

In this chapter we talk about ketosis, how to achieve it, and the science behind it. To understand how the ketogenic diet works, you should have a basic understanding of the process of ketosis. You will get an overview of what ketosis is and how inducing it will benefit you.

Ketosis is the metabolic process of converting stored fat into energy. Normally, glucose is the primary source of energy, but during ketosis, stored fat is used instead. When fats are consumed, the body is prompted to burn them for fuel because more ketones are produced in the liver, and thus the body will use fats as its prime energy source. As the body continuously needs energy, it will constantly keep burning all the extra fat stored all around your body. When this is happening, you will soon see a difference in the shape of your body and a reduction in the number on the weighing scale.

Additionally, during constant ketosis, hunger is mostly satiated, and as such, you feel fuller for longer. With time, there are fewer cravings and hunger pangs, allowing you to feel satisfied between meals. Dealing with hunger pangs is a major issue with other diets that force you to eat less. It requires a lot of will power to follow those fad diets and ignore hunger pangs.

At some point or the other, most people end up binge eating after such diets. Binge eating usually involves carbohydrate-loaded food that will cause more weight gain; however, the ketogenic diet will curb this excess hunger healthily.

During ketosis, you will feel full for longer periods even while the body is burning off excess fat. It takes a little time to adapt to the diet initially, but over time you will be able to sustain it. Another benefit is that ketosis increases the level of good cholesterol in the body, which in turn decreases the level of bad cholesterol. The HDL levels tend to rise during ketosis, and it takes the LDL for processing in the liver. HDL is essential for certain functions in your body so don't assume that all cholesterol is bad. Focus more on reducing the carbohydrates that have a negative impact on your body. Many studies have been conducted over the years to see how the ketogenic diet and ketosis affect different people. People who frequently play sports experience increased stamina and have more energy to be active for a longer period. They usually turn to carb loading for energy, but energy for carbohydrates burns off very fast. Energy derived from fats takes longer to burn and thus provides energy for a longer time. The process of ketosis also showed improvement in focus and stamina of people. Although research is still being done to study the effects and benefits of the ketogenic diet, it is one of the best ways to lose weight and get healthier.

Let us understand ketosis and its benefit in a short and simple way. We are all aware that the body uses glucose as its main source of energy for the body. When you reduce the carbohydrates in the diet and increase the fats, there isn't enough carbohydrate to use for energy. The body now needs to adapt to survive this deficit of glucose, so it will start using the fats in the body for energy. When carbohydrates are in deficit, more ketones are produced in the liver. When these ketones are used up for energy, the stored fats are then burned for energy. Thus, you will see how the ketosis process helps you burn unwanted weight off your body and get back to a healthier size. Ketosis is a natural metabolic process that works automatically when you switch to the ketogenic diet. Ketosis induces the following benefits to the body:

Reduce Appetite

Ketosis reduces appetite by One of the worst effects of fad dieting is that it leaves you very hungry and unsatisfied. This will cause you to give up quite soon and end up eating more; however, ketosis will help you in reducing your appetite itself when your carbohydrate consumption also goes down.

Weight Loss

It will help you in losing weight quite fast compared to any other method of affecting the body to burn fat. During the first week after you start following the ketogenic diet, the body will lose water weight due to low carbohydrate consumption, which also decreases insulin levels. Afterwards, fat is burned off, which results in weight loss.

Burn Abdominal Fat

Ketosis helps to burn excess abdominal fat, which is usually one of the toughest areas for fat loss. Most people spend hours at the gym doing ab exercises to lose abdominal fat, but ketosis makes this much easier. The different places that fat is stored in your body will affect your health. This abdominal fat is usually associated with insulin resistance and inflammation and can cause metabolic dysfunction. Therefore, ketosis is very beneficial for your health in getting rid of this visceral fat that lodges around the organs.

Curb Triglycerides

Triglycerides are fat molecules that circulate in the blood. Ketosis reduces the level of triglycerides very significantly. People who lead more sedentary lifestyles will tend to have increased triglycerides, which increases the risk for heart disease. Consuming a diet with too little fats will increase the level of triglycerides while a low carb diet will reduce it.

Increased Lipoproteins

Ketosis will also aid in increasing levels of high-density lipoproteins in your body. This is the good kind of cholesterol that should be there in your body and should always be higher than the bad cholesterol or LDL.

Controlling Diabetes by Reducing Insulin and Blood Pressure

Ketosis reduces blood sugar and insulin in the body. As such, ketosis helps people who suffer from diabetes type two and insulin resistance. Furthermore, ketosis can help lower high blood pressure, which is a risk factor for different diseases related to the heart and kidney.

Ketosis is also beneficial for brain health since it burns ketones. Therefore, the ketogenic diet is used to induce ketosis in children with epilepsy who might not be responding to treatment by drugs.

As you can see, there are various reasons why the ketogenic diet is used to induce ketosis in the human body. This process can have many beneficial effects on health and easily help to lose excess weight, which is detrimental to the body. We will give you a straightforward breakdown on how to achieve ketosis, consider performing the following:

First, restrict your consumption of all forms of carbohydrates.

Then, limit your intake of proteins in order to lower the level of ketosis. To lose weight, eat approximately 0.7 grams of protein per pound of your lean body mass.

You should stop worrying about and hating fat. In this diet, fats are your main source of fuel, and you should be consuming more of it without questioning yourself. Give it a chance; if you follow the guidelines given in this book, you will be burning more fat than you consume.

You must remember to drink at least a gallon of water every day in order to maintain consistent hydration, ensuring regulation of vital bodily functions and controlling hunger.

Avoid snacking in order to decrease insulin spikes throughout the day, allowing for quicker weight loss. Eating too often will slow down the process of weight loss.

Practice intermittent fasting, which fasting. In another chapter of this book, you will learn about intermittent fasting and its benefits. Fasting has been known to increase the levels of ketones in the blood.

Exercise daily for at least 30 to 40 minutes. You might start with walking to build up your stamina, aiming to achieve high-intensity workouts with time. Exercising helps to regulate blood sugar levels and aids in weight loss. Even if you reach your goal weight, continue to exercise to maintain a healthy weight and activity level.

Anti-Inflammatory Keto (30% More Effective)

Check the ingredients on the labels of any food you purchase in order to avoid unwanted carbohydrates, additives, and preservatives that are bad for your health.

Now that you've learned how to induce ketosis, keep an eye out for the following symptoms that indicate you are maintaining ketosis:

- You will notice increased urination compared to before. Keto acts like a natural diuretic that will increase the frequency of urination in your body. The acetoacetate ketone body will also be excreted in urine, and this can cause the frequency of urination.

- You might notice that your mouth has turned dry and you will feel constantly thirsty. The increased urination dehydrates the body and requires that you keep drinking enough water to replenish the electrolytes required by the body.

- One side effect of ketosis is what is known as keto breath, which results from the metabolism of acetone, a type of ketone. Acetone is found in nail polish remover, and you may find your breath smells like that for a while. Energy levels will increase while your appetite will decrease because fats take longer to metabolize, and as such, keep you energized for a longer period.

These are just some of the common symptoms that you will be able to notice over time as you continue the ketogenic diet. They will indicate that the process of ketosis is working. You do not have to stress yourself out with a lot of testing and measuring to check if you are losing weight. Trust the process and keep track of your progress to understand if you are doing something wrong. Place your focus on the nutritional part of your diet and eat the right kinds of foods within limits set by the diet in terms of macros. There is no calorie counting or portion restriction, so it is simple for anyone to follow.

Chapter 3:
The Nutritional Break Down

The following chapter will include the nutritional break down of the Keto diet, and elaborate on the percentages of fats, protein and carbohydrates that should be consumed.

The ketogenic diet reduces carbohydrate intake to the minimum amount required for good health, thus eliminating any additional adverse carbohydrates from your diet. It also increases fat consumption significantly and promotes moderate consumption of proteins, improving muscle health. The diet is more flexible than one might realize, ensuring that every individual gets the nutrition his or her body needs.

There are several variations of the ketogenic diet that can be chosen according to everyone's needs.

Standard Ketogenic Diet
Standard ketogenic diet (SKD) allows very little carbohydrate consumption with moderate amounts of protein and a high quantity of

fats. The typical breakdown is 75% fats, 20% proteins and 5% carbohydrates.

High Protein Keto

High protein ketogenic diet is, as the name indicates, includes an increased amount of proteins. The typical breakdown of this version is 60% fats, 35% proteins, and 5% carbohydrates.

Cyclical Ketogenic Diet

Cyclical ketogenic diet (CKD) allows for higher amounts of carbohydrates for a few days, followed by days of strict ketogenic diet. Typically, it includes two days of high carbohydrate intake, followed by five days of keto diet in the week.

Targeted Ketogenic Diet

Targeted ketogenic diet (TKD) is designed for people who have high levels of activity, allowing for increased carbohydrates near workout times.

If you consider the template calorie-wise, the ketogenic diet will provide 60-75% of your required calories from fats, about 15-30% of calories are sourced from proteins and carbohydrates only provide 5-10% of calories.

Usually, people who want to lose weight follow the standard ketogenic version or the high protein ketogenic diet. The other two versions are focused on accommodating the needs of athletes or as more advanced versions. The standard ketogenic version is the most highly recommended version for the user to follow. Usually, the Keto diet allows 20 to 30 grams of net carbs, but this limit can be adjusted with time. For those seeking to lose weight, it is important to keep track of the total and net carbs consumed. Net carbohydrates are the carbohydrates in food that can be digested and used for energy. Since the human body cannot digest fiber or sugar alcohols, these are not included in the calculation. The total carbohydrate count, on the other hand, includes all carbohydrates consumed. The recommended net carbohydrate limit is no more than 25 grams per day, and the total carbohydrate limit is 35 grams per day.

Proteins should be consumed according to the overall calorie requirement, and the rest of the diet should be filled with healthy fats. For instance, if your total calorie intake per day is around 1800 calories, then you must ensure that about 1300-1400 calories are in the form of fats, about 250-300 calories from proteins and the rest from carbs.

The ketogenic diet is focused on controlling the macronutrients, also known as macros, in your diet. Macros are a part of every person's diet, and they include the fats, proteins and carbohydrates. You already know the restriction placed on carbohydrate consumption and the specification for how much proteins and fats you should consume on this diet.

The exact numbers of calories can be determined by checking various factors, such as age, gender, daily activity level, body fat percentage, height, and weight. There should also be a goal, a quantifiable desired outcome that will increase motivation throughout the process. All these factors together will determine the quantity of each required macro and the other nutrients that need to be provided to their body as a part of their daily diet.

Chapter 4:
Dirty Keto

Dirty keto is a recently popularized version of the keto diet that follows the same macronutrient breakdown but is not concerned with the sources of the macronutrients. As a result, vital micronutrients that essential for good health are missing in the dirty keto diet.

The dirty keto diet does assist in weight loss, but results in unpleasant side effects, such as bloating, inflammation and hunger pangs. Once the diet is concluded, the weight returns. The dirty keto version is suitable for certain situations, such as travel, or adjusting as needed. But ultimately, the ketogenic diet with home cooking is the best healthy method to follow. If you are worried about sacrificing the variety of foods you eat outside, you will be surprised by how many keto recipes there are for you to try out. They are much healthier and will help you lose weight in the long term.

The dirty keto version of the ketogenic diet is another version you can consider. Lately, it has gained a lot of popularity because it claims to help you lose weight even while you eat junk food. Who doesn't dream of eating junk food and still staying fit? Therefore, a lot of people are trying this version of the ketogenic diet out; it is appealing to many. But there are a lot of things to consider dirty keto. Here we will weigh the pros and cons and see if you really should try this version of the diet.

The ketogenic diet minimizes carbohydrate intake and increases fat so that the body uses fats as its source of fuel. The ketogenic diet might not be a sustainable, long-term diet, although it is very beneficial for losing weight.

The dirty keto diet allows for binge eating junk food for meals if the carbohydrate content is kept at a minimum. As a result, you may not be obtaining the necessary nutrients, healthy fats and macronutrients your body requires. People may end up eating a lot of butter, bacon, cheese and other foods that are technically keto-friendly as they are high in fats; but they are also high in cholesterol and can have a negative impact on your health. Excessive consumptions of such food can significantly increase the risk of heart diseases.

Some versions of dirty keto meals include steaks smothered with butter, mounds of cheddar cheese on enchiladas that are low in carbs, etc. You might lose weight when you switch to this dirty keto version, but it is an unhealthy choice. You will be consuming only unhealthy food as your meal replacements, and these will have no health benefits other than losing weight. The term "dirty keto" is just another way to refer to the fast and dirty way of eating packaged and processed foods instead of wholesome home-cooked meals. The only advantage of the dirty keto diet is that it is convenient.

The ketogenic diet already removes carbohydrates in a major way from your diet. When you switch to dirty keto, you will also be removing all the healthy foods that will sustain your body and keep it in good form for a long time. Sole focus on macronutrients from the dirty keto diet will result in a deficiency of nutrients that are nourishing for your gut. Your digestive system requires certain resistant starches, prebiotic fibers, etc. that are only supplied when you eat a healthy planned diet that contains the required components like vegetables. These are essential for good gut health, and if you neglect them, you will surely see the detrimental effects it has on your health. The keto diet ensures a holistic approach to food that ensures all the nutrients your body needs are met, while the dirty keto diet usually results in deficiencies due to the lack of focus and thoughtful consideration of meals. The dirty keto diet often contains foods high in saturated fats, which are pro-inflammatory and linked to hearts diseases and diabetes. The usual ketogenic diet will encourage you to eat vegetables and starchy food that is healthy for you; however, all these components are removed in the dirty keto version. It won't benefit you to substitute buns for some lettuce in your burger. You are still only eating junk food that does not provide nutrients to your diet. The clean keto diet will help you cook with healthy fats like coconut oil, olive oil or butter but in the dirty keto diet, you will be wallowing in pork rinds.

Despite such factors, a lot of people would prefer to try the dirty keto diet to lose weight. The dirty keto diet tends to be more appealing because it can be very difficult to make permanent and real changes in diet and lifestyle, requiring effort and self-education. It has much easier rules to follow, and allows for junk food, and as a result, it only achieves short-term gains at the best, with no move towards a long-term healthy body and lifestyle. This is where you must decide if you want the long-term benefits of the standard ketogenic diet or the short-term weight loss benefits of the dirty keto diet.

The regular or clean keto diet will provide you with 5% calories from carbs, 75-90% calories from fats and 6-25% calories from fats. The numbers can be adjusted within these given ranges. But the dirty keto diet does not include any specifications to determine and ensure you have obtained the required macronutrients and there are no guidelines for healthy food suggestions. You can go to any fast food restaurant and simply opt out of the carbohydrate ingredients. Dirty keto can be a very tempting alternative for those who love fast food or hate to cook. It can be an option when you occasionally eat out to choose such dirty keto friendly options; however, if you eat junk food for all your meals, your system will suffer. However, the quality of the food you eat is more important than eating for the sake of eating or losing weight; the quality of food directly impacts your health. Therefore, the dirty keto version is not what anyone would recommend for long-term use. You need to think carefully about your diet and make sure it contains all the required sources of fiber, minerals, vitamins, etc.

When you try the ketogenic diet, you should opt for the version that is clean, holistic and recommends healthy foods while removing processed, unhealthy products.

Dairy and Meats in Keto

A lot of people wonder if they should eat dairy products or meat during a ketogenic diet. Some dairy foods and meat are keto friendly while others are not and should be reduced or eliminated. The food and quantity will be determined by your body, goals, and factors such as lactose intolerance.

With regards to dairy foods, products like condensed milk or yogurts that have sugar added are not keto-friendly. Instead, you could eat ghee, butter, and hard cheeses. Certain foods that have a lot of fats are ideal for keto diet. Ghee and butter can be used for cooking since they are nearly exclusively composed of fat. For those who are lactose intolerant, ghee is a suitable alternative to butter. If your aim is to lose weight, you will simply have to monitor how much ghee or butter you consume.

In considering cheeses, certain types are much lower in carbohydrates and are thus keto-friendly. However, the exact type of cheese should be considered in order to determine the specific macros, and thus overall benefit. Typically, parmesan, gouda, brie, goat cheese, mozzarella, feta, and cheddar varieties are quite low in carbohydrates. Avoid specialty cheeses that have added ingredients such as fruit, which are quite high in carbohydrates. Generally, if you don't over-indulge on cheese, it is usually a keto-friendly ingredient.

As an ingredient, milk can be substituted with heavy cream (the better option) or half and half in desserts or coffees. These dairy products are more keto-friendly than milk since they contain a relatively low amount of carbohydrates. Try to use real heavy cream, which is about 40% fat and unsweetened. However, if you have a serious dairy intolerance, cut them out of your diet.

In dairy products, fat can range from no fat (0%) to total fat (100%). Fat can be saturated or unsaturated; note that some foods can contain both, forming a complex form of natural fat, which can benefit your health. Dairy products also contain many micronutrients like vitamin D, vitamin B12, and calcium, which are required by the body.

When you are trying to lose weight, it might help to cut down on dairy products and tracking your consumption since they are very easy to overeat and as a result, cause significant weight gain if consumed in excess. If you are facing difficulty in adapting to fat as your body's main source of fuel, or you've reached a plateau in weight loss, you might consider going dairy-free for a while. You should also consider it if you want to balance some autoimmune condition or have digestive issues such as diarrhea.

Anti-Inflammatory Keto (30% More Effective)

Ultimately, most dairy products are keto-friendly, so you can continue eating them in healthy versions of food. Don't overload on cheese if you are on a dirty keto diet since it will just make you gain more weight.

Now let's talk about meat. Usually, most diets will instruct you to opt for leaner meats such as chicken breast, and you are expected to give up fatty steaks and pork. The keto diet does not impose this restriction, but rather encourages greasy meats in moderation. Meat contains a lot of protein, which can take you out of the state of ketosis that the ketogenic diet aims to induce. Therefore, you cannot have a very meat heavy keto diet. They are okay to consume in moderation, but they should not be a staple in your everyday meals.

The leaner cuts of meat that other diets recommend include chicken breasts, but these are very high in protein. If you want to achieve ketosis, you cannot eat too much proteins. The main reason is that the body converts protein into glucose through a process called gluconeogenesis, which means that eating high amounts of protein will increase your body's glucose levels. This would be counterproductive to the ketogenic diet and will prevent ketosis. Your body will use the protein for glucose and then the glucose for energy. The fats will stay stored and will add to your weight. Therefore, on the keto diet, only one-fifth of your meal should consist of protein. Therefore, incorporate mostly non-meat sources of fat in your meals in order to avoid gluconeogenesis. This does not mean you cannot eat meats; however, do so sparingly. In terms of good fat to protein ratio, the meats that are allowed include fatty steaks, such as ribeye and brisket, unprocessed and nitrate-free bacon, chicken thighs with skin, fatty fish like salmon, and organ meats like liver or heart. Be sure to consider the protein content and omit them from your regular diet. Instead opt for animal fats such as lard or bacon grease, ghee, and eggs.

Chapter 5:
The Mediterranean Diet

In this chapter, we will discuss what the Mediterranean diet is and how it will benefit your health.

The Mediterranean diet is a very heart-healthy diet plan that is based on recipes from Mediterranean cuisine. It comprises of foods that people from countries around the Mediterranean, such as Italy, Greece eat. Research has shown that their diets were exceptionally healthy with minimal reported diseases that are prevalent these days and are related specifically to food and lifestyle. The studies also show that the Mediterranean diet aids in weight loss, and can reduce the risk of heart diseases, Type 2 diabetes, and even premature death.

The diet incorporates basic healthy eating practices alongside olive oil or red wine added to the meal. These are just some of the components that characterize Mediterranean cooking and make it flavorfull yet healthy. Although all healthy diets recommend nearly the same wholesome fruit, vegetables, whole grains, certain subtle variations make a difference. This variation seems to contribute to decreased levels of LDL and reduces the risk of heart diseases, cancer, Alzheimer's and Parkinson's diseases, and breast cancer. This diet helps to lower the level of LDL or bad cholesterol that is likely to build up in your arteries and cause issues. The Mediterranean diet is also not limited to one type of food or one form of cuisine. It encompasses many countries that surround the Mediterranean Sea, and thus you get to try a wide variety of dishes to select from. The Mediterranean diet is characterized by a high intake of plant-based foods, olive oil, moderate consumption of fish or poultry, and relatively low intake of dairy, red meats, sweets, and processed foods. Red wine is consumed in moderation as an accompaniment to a meal and is considered beneficial to the heart. There is a strong focus on communal meals in which everyone eats together, emphasizing the social and cultural aspects of the society. They also tend to rest after meals and are quite active on a regular basis. Due to westernization, however, there has been an increase in processed food within the Mediterranean countries, contributing to increased health concerns.

In the Mediterranean lifestyle, daily physical activity also plays an important role. It helps to maintain and attain the overall good health of every individual. You can try some regular running or aerobics or other activities that are more leisurely such as walking or just taking the stairs. Another easy way to stay active is to do some physical work around the house like cleaning or yard work. Anything that keeps you moving and active will benefit your health and especially your heart health. It will also aid in losing weight over time.

The Mediterranean diet is not just another hype diet and has scientific evidence to prove that it is beneficial for health. It is known to lower mortality, morbidity, cancer risk, cardiovascular disease, obesity, cognitive disease, metabolic syndrome, etc. Studies also show that patterns of the Mediterranean diet can help in the prevention or control of non-communicable diseases that are related to diet. The better the knowledge and access to healthy food, the higher the chances of the person staying disease free. According to the Mediterranean diet, you should emphasize the following:

- Eat more plant-based foods like vegetables, fruit, whole grains, nuts and legumes
- Use canola oil or olive oil instead of butter
- Eat fish or poultry about two times a week
- Use herbs and spices instead of salt to flavor food
- Eat red meat no more than two times a month
- Eat meals with family and friends
- Accompany your meal with a glass of red wine
- Exercise regularly

- Don't eat processed foods, added sugars, or refined grains
- Avoid trans fats from margarine or other processed foods
- Avoid low fat, diet and processed foods

Foods Found in the Mediterranean Diet

Traditionally, the Mediterranean diet includes a lot of fruit, rice, vegetables and pasta with fewer animal-sourced foods. The Mediterranean diet includes:

- Vegetables: tomatoes, broccoli, spinach, onions, cauliflower, cucumbers, kale, etc.
- Fruit: apples, bananas, melons, peaches, figs, dates, grapes, etc.
- Nuts: almonds, hazelnuts, walnuts, etc.
- Seeds: pumpkin seeds, sunflower seeds, etc.
- Legumes: beans, pulses (i.e. dried seeds of legumes), peanuts, peas, etc.
- Tubers: turnips, sweet potatoes, potatoes, etc.
- Eggs: chicken, duck or quail.
- Whole grains: brown rice, rye, corn, buckwheat, whole oats, etc.
- Fish or seafood: crab, trout, salmon, shrimp, oysters, etc.

- Poultry: duck, turkey or chicken.

- Dairy: cheese, Greek yogurt, etc.

- Herbs and spices: nutmeg, mint, rosemary, pepper and cinnamon.

- Healthy fats from avocados, olives, olive oil, etc.

- Water to stay hydrated.

- Tea and coffee (as you want without added sugars) and avoiding processed juices and beverages.

Benefits of The Mediterranean Diet

The Mediterranean diet is a healthy and nutritious diet that improves your quality of life and wellbeing without placing any extreme limits on your diet and allowing you to continue enjoying delicious foods. As you adapt to Mediterranean dietary habits, you will soon notice the benefits it has on your heart, brain, and overall health and longevity. Following are elaborations on some of the benefits of the Mediterranean diet on your body and mind:

Reduces the Risk of Type 2 Diabetes.

Many studies have demonstrated that the Mediterranean diet is highly beneficial for those who with diabetes or high blood pressure because it emphasizes foods with more monounsaturated fats and fiber. As a result, blood sugar levels and cholesterol decrease, aiding in the management of Type 2 diabetes. Replacing saturated or trans fats with unsaturated fats also assist in regulating insulin sensitivity.

Improves Heart Health

The incidence of heart diseases is low in Mediterranean countries compared to the United States, mainly due to the difference in dietary choices and activity level. They also drink a glass of red wine daily, and this also benefits heart health.

Maintains Agility with Age

Since this diet provides your body with all the nutrients it requires, alongside physical activity, there is a reduction in the risk of muscle weakness and frailty that occur with age. This diet has shown to reduce this risk of weakening muscles by more than half in people above 60. +

Reduces the Risk of Parkinson's Disease

The Mediterranean diet incorporates high amounts of antioxidants, which can reduce the risk of Parkinson's disease. These antioxidants are obtained from the fresh fruits and vegetables, seafood and healthy fat sources. Furthermore, antioxidants protect cells from oxidative stress, which can cause damage and promote the development of Parkinson's disease. Oxidation is a very common process that takes place in the body. On the other hand, oxidative stress occurs due to an imbalance between antioxidants and free radicals present in the body. When the body is functioning optimally, then these free radicals help fight off pathogens. When the number of free radical's present exceeds the number of antioxidants present, then the free radicals start to damage the DNA, proteins and other fatty tissues within the body. All this can lead to several illnesses over time if left unchecked.

Reduces the Risk of Alzheimer's Disease

As a result of the diet contributing to decreased cholesterol and blood sugar levels, the overall health of blood vessels improves, therefore reducing the risk of Alzheimer's, dementia, and other cognitive impairments. In this way, the quality of life can be preserved due to limited occurrences of burdensome illnesses.

Encourages Healthy Weight Loss

One primary advantage of the Mediterranean diet is that it is very easy to maintain long-term since it is not unreasonably restrictive and allows you to eat enough to satisfy your hunger, and thus stay satiated longer. The addition of regular exercise will allow you to lose weight steadily over time in a way that can be managed more easily for a longer period of time, which is a part of the Mediterranean lifestyle, and so you will see major weight loss if you stick to the diet for a longer time. Diets that allow you to lose weight too quickly are usually unhealthy and not sustainable. The Mediterranean diet encourages the body to slowly but steadily lose unhealthy weight in a way that can be managed for the long term.

Helps Fight Cancer

Research has shown that the Mediterranean diet can reduce the risk of cancer from developing, as well as cancer-related mortality. There seems to be some probable protective role against cancer that is played by the Mediterranean diet. More specifically, this diet is considered helpful in the prevention of the occurrence of breast cancer in women post menopause. This is especially beneficial since this breast cancer usually has a poor prognosis.

Maintains Cognitive Health

It is considered that following the Mediterranean diet will reduce the risk of development of degenerative diseases like Parkinson's or dementia. Studies have indicated that following this diet can improve a person's cognitive abilities by enhancing memory and improving focus and attention. This diet is also considered beneficial for progressing the language capabilities of the brain, which can assist in preventing dementia as well as maintaining general healthy brain function. This will help in better performance at work, better mental health and overall improvement in the quality of life.

Encourages Relaxation

The Mediterranean diet is not just a meal plan but a lifestyle. The meals are a very social experience, with a lot of time spent outside or exercising in one way or another. This lifestyle improves stress management and relaxation, allowing them to sleep better, have more energy and form better relationships.

Improves Mood Swings

Hectic and unhealthy lifestyles often cause mental health issues like depression, anxiety and mood swings. The Mediterranean diet has shown to have brain-boosting effects that help alleviate such symptoms and improve mental health. When the brain doesn't have enough dopamine hormone, these disorders tend to occur since this hormone is responsible for mood regulation, thought processing and body movements. The healthy foods encouraged by this diet ensure enough production of this chemical so that your mood remains elevated and happy. It also contributes to good gut health, which is also linked to mood triggers. Mental health disorders require proper treatment, but the diet acts as an effective aid for prevention as well as control.

Helps Fight Inflammation

The Mediterranean diet has been shown to reduce and regulate inflammation in the body, as well as any conditions that might arise from chronic inflammation. Oxidative stress is a major trigger for inflammation, but it can be reduced with antioxidants. If you eat more of foods containing choline, then you can further increase this positive impact Consuming more egg yolks, soybean, beets, and spinach will help to reduce inflammation.

Improves Skin

Your skin is highly impacted by your diet, so many doctors will recommend diet changes for people suffering from various skin conditions. The olive oil used in Mediterranean cooking contains a lot of vitamin E and antioxidants, which help to hydrate and nourish the skin. Red wine also contains resveratrol, which inhibits the growth of acne-causing bacteria. Another staple in the Mediterranean diet is tomato, which protects skin cells from cancer caused by exposure to the sun's ultraviolet rays.

Helps Relieve Pain

Since the Mediterranean diet consists of foods such as whole grains that are rich in magnesium, as well as fruit and vegetables that are rich in fiber, it naturally provides a means to assist in pain management, especially for those who suffer from chronic pain. This diet reduces inflammation, which can make a big difference in managing and reducing, and as such, alleviating stress. To benefit more from this pain-relieving aspect, you should increase your intake of foods that are rich in magnesium as it is proven to fight muscle pain. So, try to eat more of nuts, seeds, leafy greens, lentils, whole grains and beans.

Benefit Fertility

Studies showed that women who followed the Mediterranean diet were more fertile than women who followed a normal balanced diet and even demonstrated higher fertility after they switched to this diet. This diet can also benefit men in developing healthier sperm to increase likelihood of conception.

Increases Longevity

Anti-Inflammatory Keto (30% More Effective)

Between 1960 and 1990, mortality statistics showed that the people who lived in the Mediterranean region lived longer and the major contributing factor for this was their diet. The Mediterranean lifestyle can help you live longer, healthier and happier when all the aspects of their daily life are adapted.

Chapter 6:
Ketogenic Mediterranean Diet

In this chapter, you will learn how to combine the ketogenic diet with the Mediterranean diet. Both the diet's benefits that can easily assist any individual in losing weight and improving overall health by developing a more nutritious diet and active lifestyle.

The Mediterranean diet is a very widely accepted nutritional regime due to its evident health benefits from the macronutrient composition of the food and the active lifestyle. These contribute significantly to the health of the people who consume the Mediterranean diet, and thus they benefit from the most health benefits possible.

When it comes to losing weight, the ketogenic diet is a viable option to achieve any set weight goals. The ketogenic diet has a strong basis both physiologically and biochemically, allowing it to be useful for weight loss and heart health. Merging the ketogenic diet with the Mediterranean diet can have some of the best possible outcomes for someone who practices it appropriately.

Anti-Inflammatory Keto (30% More Effective)

Solely following the ketogenic diet often results in an imbalanced intake of fats due to the increased consumption of trans fats, saturated fats, or omega6 acids., and not enough intake of monosaturated fats and omega-3 fatty acids that are good for heart health.

By itself, the ketogenic diet inadvertently causes a heightened focus on macronutrients and too little focus on the micronutrients. When the food quality and micronutrient density is not enough or appropriate, you may face issues like hormone dysregulation, inflammation, and weight stalls. It also does not incorporate foods such as non-starchy vegetables, fatty fish, and virgin olive oil, which are included in the Mediterranean diet. The nutrient density, and active lifestyle of the Mediterranean diet can be combined with the standard ketogenic diet to lose weight and maximize health benefits.

Merging the two diets together will consist of olive oil, green vegetables, avocados, coconut oil, fish, eggs, cheese and lean meat, and a moderate consumption of red wine. Whole grains, starchy vegetables like potatoes, corn or peas, legumes and any food containing sugar or flour are eliminated.

The Keto-Mediterranean diet does not include fruit, even though it is a healthy food choice, due to the sugar fruits contain. The main emphasis is on using olive oil, fish, healthier fat and red wine. These are the few essential components that are common to the diet of all the people around the Mediterranean region. This is what differentiates this diet from other forms of the keto diet. A lot of evidence has demonstrated that combining the two diets can be very effective in reducing unhealthy appetites and unwanted weight, as well as being beneficial for people who suffer from heart disease, diabetes, and epilepsy. The Keto-Mediterranean diet can also help to reduce fasting glucose levels, prevent insulin resistance, cholesterol and triglycerides.

Olive oil is the main component of the Mediterranean diet that should be included in your diet due to its health benefits. Olive oil reduces the risk associated with most cardiovascular disease by influencing factors such as lipoprotein profile, glucose metabolism and blood pressure. It also reduces inflammation, oxidative stress and endothelial function. These positive effects are usually attributed to the monounsaturated fatty acids found within oil olive, especially extra virgin olive oil. Compounds like hydrocarbons, sterols, and polyphenols have demonstrated antioxidant, anti-inflammatory and even hypolipidemic properties. Studies have shown that a diet that is rich in monounsaturated fats will prevent both central fat redistribution and insulin resistance that is usually induced when the diet is rich in carbohydrates.

Red wine consists of phenolic compounds (this lends certain foods their red color) and ethanol, and these phenolic compounds are what contribute to the associated protection against cardiovascular diseases. Consuming red wine is beneficial due to the antiatherogenic properties of the antioxidant polyphenols. This combination also has a positive effect on hemodynamics. The amount of wine that should be consumed, if at all, varies with everyone, who should consult with his or her doctor first.

Fish contain three active components: docosahexaenoic acid, eicosatetraenoic acid, and two long chain omega-3 PUFA. Studies have shown that people who consume a lot of fish in their diets have lower rates of coronary heart disease. However, the consumption of fish should be limited as they may contain high levels of mercury, which is harmful to human health. Large fish with longer lifespans, like sharks or swordfish, have higher concentrations of omega-3 in their tissues, whereas smaller fish lower concentrations. The high concentration of omega 3 in fish helps increase insulin sensitivity and reduce inflammation. Saturated fats have a higher tendency to get stored as fat in the body while mono or polyunsaturated fats are more effectively used in fat oxidation.

Generally, people have the misconception that eating more fats and protein in their diet will cause excessive weight gain; however, studies conducted with the ketogenic Mediterranean diet proved that this diet is very effective in reducing weight and dealing with obesity. Unlike most other diets, the Keto-Mediterranean diet does not impose any calorie restrictions, although it does recommend avoiding overeating. The reason behind this effectiveness of the ketogenic Mediterranean diet is the synergy between the high protein keto nature and the MUFA (Monounsaturated fats) as well as PUFA (Polyunsaturated fats) in the Mediterranean diet. A lot of studies have confirmed that compared to other conventional low carbohydrate diets, the ketogenic diet is much more effective in treating obesity. A diet with high-unsaturated fat is also quite effective in preserving lean mass compared to a diet that is low in fats or carbohydrates. Studies also demonstrated that the ketogenic Mediterranean diet improves fasting glycemic index quite significantly. Since the diet also significantly reduced total cholesterol, LDL cholesterol, triacylglycerol's, etc. it creates a very positive cardiovascular profile. Red wine plays an important role in this last point as it also helps to increase levels of good cholesterol or HDL. Ultimately, you can see that all the factors of the ketogenic as well as the Mediterranean diet play an important role in the overall improvement of health and not just in losing weight. It is important to remember that the Mediterranean lifestyle plays a crucial role and not the just the food so imbibing it into your daily life would also be important if you were to follow the ketogenic Mediterranean diet.

As you read on, you will learn more about what foods you should or should not eat in the Ketogenic Mediterranean diet. The following are some tips to help you in the process of switching to this diet.

Reduce or eliminate the "white" foods, such as bread, pasta, cereals, rice and potatoes, because they all refined foods filled with starchy carbohydrates. Instead, switch to beans, lentil, and quinoa since these are healthy and quite filling as well. Also, limit the consumption of brown rice although it does not have to be eliminated.

Completely eliminate any sugar, sweetened drinks, and other sweetened foods because it is not beneficial to your health and mainly has adverse effects, such as weight gain, obesity and diabetes. There are a lot of keto-friendly desserts that you can opt for instead.

Consume as many vegetables as you can, adding a variety of colors on your plate, especially dark, leafy greens. Eat non-starchy vegetables as they will help increase your vital phytonutrient consumption. Phytonutrients are certain compounds that are essential to keep your body working properly and there are more than 25,000 types of phytonutrients present in plant-based foods. However, the most important of all are carotenoids, ellagic acid, flavonoids, resveratrol, phytoestrogens and glycosylates. By consuming keto-friendly plant-based produce, your body will be able to obtain all these necessary phytonutrients. There are a variety of recipes that you can try to make your meals healthy and delicious at the same time while using these ingredients.

Regularly add at least one to two ounces of a high-quality protein sources in your diet because your body requires a constant intake of protein since it is not stored internally. This will help you prevent muscle loss and reduce unhealthy appetites. Limit your consumption of processed meats. High-quality sources of protein include seafood, soy, oily fish, meat, tofu, chickpeas, lentils, nuts, and quinoa.

Eat one portion of fruit per day instead of processed or unhealthy snacks. You may select options like berries and pears. You should eat the fruits with edible peels since that is where most of the nutrients lie. Reduce intake of tropical fruits that are high in sugar, such as mangoes and bananas.

Don't cut out full-fat dairy products from your diet. There is a misguided fear that they are not good for your health or weight, but in fact, it is the opposite. You may even eat dairy such as cheese that might be high in calories, since it will keep you full for longer and provide fuel for energy.

Consume healthy fats and oils, like olive oil, in order to improve the absorption of essential fat-soluble vitamins.

Add vinegar to your diet because it can help in the process of weight loss, burning off abdominal fat, improving insulin sensitivity, and reducing blood sugar spikes after meals.

Stay hydrated by drinking plenty of water. There is no fixed quantity of water that everyone must drink, and while some should drink more, others might require less water for good health. Keep your body size, metabolic rate and rate of daily activity in mind as you determine your appropriate water content.

Anti-Inflammatory Keto (30% More Effective)

Save desserts for special occasions, and don't overindulge.

Control your portion size during meals so that you don't overeat. You could eat five small meals in a day rather than three larger meals; this is helpful because frequent meals can help curb unhealthy cravings. You can still stick to the breakfast-lunch-dinner routine but eat just enough to satiate your appetite. If you are hungry between meals, eat small portions of some keto-friendly snacks.

Studies show that people who strictly follow the Ketogenic Mediterranean diet have a significantly lower body mass index. It is an effective alternative to low-fat diets that are usually followed but don't work. This diet also has a much better effect on glycemic control and the lipids in the body.

Although there is no limit on calorie intake, moderation is key if you want to lose excess weight. Eating excessively will always cause weight gain regardless of the diet you follow and will strain your digestive system. This does not mean you can't have a slice of birthday cake at a party, but you should limit the size and minimize intake. You can always have a glass of wine or a pint of beer with your friends but limit it to no more than two. As we said, moderation will play an important role while you still enjoy a delicious and healthy diet.

If you are following the Ketogenic Mediterranean diet to lose or maintain weight, visit a doctor or professional to determine what your healthy weight range is. This range is determined based on your height, age, and overall health, and should be your guide. If your current weight is above the recommended healthy weight range, then you may have to put extra effort in cutting back on extra food, as well as adding more exercise into your daily routine.

Since the Keto-Mediterranean diet does not require counting calories, you shouldn't experience pressure, and hopefully will be more likely to succeed. Thankfully, this diet does not require any such thing, and thus you will feel less likely to fail. Just follow the guidelines given in this book and practice moderation. This will help you to lose your excess weight and stay healthy in the long term. In the case of pregnant women or children, we recommend consultation from a doctor to determine what the exact dietary requirements are for optimum health.

Chapter 7:
Keto-Mediterranean Vegetables

The Keto-Mediterranean diet features a variety of ingredients from all around the Mediterranean Sea that can be easily adaptable to your daily meals.

Vegetables should be eaten with every meal since they are very important sources of vitamins, fiber, nutrients, minerals and antioxidants. They are also great snacks to maintain satiety between meals and can be drizzled with or cooked in olive oil. You even have the option of having delicious raw vegetables for instance in a healthy salad. For a keto Mediterranean diet. The vegetables you select should be low in carbohydrate content, so avoid starchy vegetables like potatoes. Instead, you have a wide variety of good keto-friendly vegetables to choose from which have been a part of the Mediterranean diet for years together.

Some of the recommended vegetables in the Mediterranean diet are listed below:

Artichokes

You can enjoy the soft, deep and subtle flavors of this incredible green by steaming it. This vegetable is rich in magnesium, iron, vitamin C, and antioxidants, and it has prebiotic properties as well. So, this helps improve your gut's health.

Arugula
The peppery flavor and aroma of arugula adds a wonderful texture to a salad. This vegetable is rich in chlorophyll and helps to prevent DNA and liver damage caused by aflatoxins. Aflatoxins are certain harmful carcinogens that are produced by specific molds that grow in soil and decaying vegetables and grains.

Beets
Beets, also known as beetroots, are vegetables rich in manganese, folate, and iron, and are packed with essential minerals, vitamins and plant compounds with medicinal properties. Beets taste delicious and are extremely easy to add to your diet.

Cabbage
Cabbages are often overlooked although they are packed with nutrients and are rich in antioxidants that help prevent inflammation. .

Brussels Sprouts
Brussels sprouts resemble a mini cabbage and are packed with nutrients, antioxidants and fiber.

Celery

Celery is a crispy and crunchy vegetable that is low in calories, rich in antioxidants, and aids in digestion.

Chicory
The chicory root is a food additive found in a variety of products, like in coffee and as a food additive. This root is rich in dietary fiber, which is soluble in insulin. Dietary fiber helps reduce the absorption of carbs and this in turn reduces the blood glucose and insulin levels. The reduction of these levels in helpful while fighting obesity and diabetes.

Cucumbers
Cucumber is a fruit. It is low in calories and has large amounts of water and dietary fiber, aiding in weight loss and increasing hydration.

Eggplant
Eggplants have a toothsome texture and very neutral flavor, making it very suitable for sauces quite nicely. This vegetable can also be used to mimic meat. It is a nutritional powerhouse with fiber and potassium. A concentrated compound in the skin called chlorogenic acid also has anti-viral and anti-cancer properties.

Fennel
Fennel is packed with copper, zinc, calcium, potassium, vitamin C, selenium, manganese, magnesium and iron. Fennel seeds are packed

with nutrients that assist in water retention and regulating blood pressure.

Mustard Greens

Mustard greens are loaded with nutrients that ward off diseases. They have a rich, peppery flavor and are so light in calories that you can eat as much as you want.

Mushrooms

Mushrooms are a type of fungi, and are rich in protein, fiber, and antioxidants.

Kale

Kale is one of the most nutritious leafy greens loaded with nutrients and antioxidants, and it can help lower cholesterol.

Leeks

Leeks are sweet and can be eaten cooked or raw. This vegetable has antimicrobial properties and is rich in antioxidants.

Bell Peppers

Peppers can be eaten in any way, such as fresh, ground, or roasted, and are rich sources of vitamin A, and vitamin C. They also contain folate, fiber, beta-carotene and some vitamin K. Red peppers contain lycopene and lutein, which aid infighting macular degeneration.

Anti-Inflammatory Keto (30% More Effective)

These are many more vegetables available that you can choose from for your Keto-friendly Mediterranean meals. They can all be cooked or consumed in a variety of ways, keeping your meals appetizing and healthy. Other vegetables you can eat include turnips, zucchini, onions, radishes, peas, okra, broccoli, scallions, and spinach.

Chapter 8:
Keto Mediterranean Meats and Nuts

In this chapter, we will talk about Mediterranean foods in the form of fish, meats, nuts, and beans, that are keto friendly and can be a part of your diet. These are all foods that can easily be found and thus made a part of your meals. These foods have been consumed as a part of the daily diets of the people who live in the countries around the Mediterranean Sea and are their main source of protein. It is important to provide your body with some good protein even when you are trying to lose weight. It plays an important role in your body and prevents muscle wasting as well. As you read on you will understand why we recommend these foods and why they are an important part of your diet.

Let's first start with fish since they are the best source of protein in the Mediterranean diet, rather than other meats. Consumption of fish that is rich in omega-3 fats is considered one of the healthiest aspects of the Keto-Mediterranean diet. This includes fish like wild salmon, which is quite oily. A study published in the Nutrition Research journal in 2016 showed that overweight men or women who started consuming salmon a couple of times a week saw improvement in their blood fat profile.

The more fish is consumed, the better its health benefits. Consuming salmon aids in reducing triglycerides in the blood and increases HDL cholesterol levels. There is also a positive impact on lipoprotein molecule sizes, which is important as it helps to reduce the risk of coronary artery disease. A diet that includes salmon will be very good for the health of the heart. It is recommended to consume ocean fish or wild fish instead of farmed fish, if possible. The former contains more levels of omega-3 fatty acids that are beneficial for health. You also should be careful about consuming too much tuna or swordfish because these types of fish can contain high levels of mercury, that is very toxic when it builds up. A lot of people suffer from mercury toxicity due to over-consumption of these fish so you should consume them sparingly. The Keto-Mediterranean diet recommends fish as a part of your diet 2-3 times a week. Include fish that contain low levels of mercury such as sardines, salmon, flounder, shrimp, crab, lobster or cod. Limit the consumption of bluefish, tuna, Chilean sea bass, swordfish, halibut or grouper. These types of fish will increase oxidative stress in your body and reduce intracellular glutathione. To counter mercury toxicity, you can inquire about selenium supplements.

Some years ago, people started discouraging the consumption of nuts because these are high in fat; however, the Keto-Mediterranean diet prompts you to consume nuts in your diet for the very same reason and emphasizes that they are healthy. You should be careful and consume a limited amount, but there is no reason to cut them out of your diet completely. Nuts are healthy ingredients that can reduce the risk of cancer, cardiovascular diseases, as well as increase longevity. Studies were conducted to compare those who consumed a limited quantity of nuts every day to those who did not. The research showed that the ones who consumed nuts had a significantly lower risk of heart diseases. The European Journal of Nutrition also published a study that said walnuts, peanuts and other such nuts helped to reduce weight and prevention of obesity. This is because the nuts are very low in carbohydrates and rich in fiber.

Another study conducted and published in the New England Journal of Medicine stated that amongst people with a high risk of cardiovascular diseases, those who consumed a Mediterranean diet were at much lower risk, demonstrating that the diet actually reduces the chances of many illnesses, slows down the aging process and also increases life expectancy.

The following are some of the nuts, beans, legumes and seeds, and seafood that can be included in the Ketogenic Mediterranean diet. You will also learn of some of their benefits and why you should consume them.

Almonds

They are a rich source of vitamin E, healthy fats, protein and other minerals. Almonds are considered helpful in lowering blood sugar levels, blood pressure and high cholesterol. They also aid in reducing cravings and thus promote weight loss. They contain many bioactive molecules that can help in the prevention of cardiovascular diseases.

Cashews

A lot of people avoid this nut because they think it will make them fat; however, cashews can have a lot of health benefits and should be added to your diet in a limited quantity. They are high in fat and are also a good source of vitamin E and minerals like zinc and magnesium. They also aid in boosting the immune system and have anti-cancerous properties.

Hazelnuts

Hazelnuts are very common in the region of Italy and can be eaten as snacks, used in sauces, or added on as a garnish to your dish. They contain a lot of monounsaturated fat and are a good source of vitamin E, folate, protein, calcium and fiber. It also contains arginine, which is beneficial for the blood vessels.

Pistachios

Pistachios are very rich in nutrient and taste delicious. They aid in digestion and help to control diabetes. Pistachios are considered helpful in the management of weight and reduce bad LDL cholesterol levels. They are rich in antioxidants and contribute to skin hydration. They can also reduce the risk of macular disease related to age.

Walnuts

They contain MUFA and PUFA, which are the healthy fats your diet needs. They are a super source of omega-3 fatty acids, as well as iron, selenium, zinc and calcium. They promote a healthy gut and help lower blood pressure. They are also used in the management of Type 2 Diabetes and reduce inflammation.

Pine Nuts

They contribute to good heart health and are a great source of monounsaturated fatty acids. Pine nuts can help lower LDL and the risk of heart attacks. They have a light taste and texture that makes them a great ingredient in salads.

Split Peas

They provide vitamin K, which promotes the heart as well as bone health. They also contain thiamine and fiber, which helps in blood sugar management and supporting brain health. They are very rich sources of minerals for your diet.

Kidney Beans

Kidney beans are a power-packed source of proteins and minerals. They lower cholesterol levels and are a good ingredient for people with diabetes. They are considered helpful in losing weight and promote good colon health. They have detoxifying properties and boost energy. Kidney beans are also said to aid in the prevention of hypertension and memory retention.

Fava Beans

These beans are dense with nutrition and contain no saturated fat. They help in the treatment of Parkinson's disease symptoms and reduce symptoms of anemia too. They contain a high amount of thiamine, vitamin B6 and K, copper, magnesium and selenium. They also boost the immune system and can help in the prevention of congenital disabilities.

Sesame Seeds

They are rich in polyunsaturated fatty acids as well as omega-3 fatty acids. They are good for skin and hair health. They also boost energy levels and promote bone health. The magnesium content in sesame seeds is considered helpful in preventing hypertension.

Chickpeas

If you eat them daily, chickpeas provide protein, folate, calcium, iron and zinc. They are also a good source of soluble and insoluble fibers that will keep you full for longer periods. Chickpeas also have phytate and phytosterols and can help manage diabetes or reducing the risk of heart disease or colon cancer.

Lentils

They are very low in calories and are a great source of iron, folate and protein. They have a high content of polyphenols that promote good health and reduce the risk of heart diseases. The complex carbs in lentils help to boost metabolism and aid the process of burning fats. The fiber in lentils reduces cholesterol levels in the blood.

The following are some of the fish and meats that you should include in your diet. You can eat them for lunch or dinner a couple of times a week. Try to consume more of fish than meat, as they are a good source of omega-3 fatty acids that will benefit your heart. People in the Mediterranean countries tend to eat meat in very small portions, and more often than naught prefer lean cuts. Poultry is one of the better sources of lean protein since it does not have the high amount of saturated fats that can be found in some red meats.

Abalone
Abalones can be eaten raw or cooked, taste great either way. They are a great source of vital nutrients and are especially beneficial for eye and skin health. They are low in fat and provide omega-3 fatty acids to your diet.

Clams
Clams are a nutritious food with many health benefits. You get lean protein, minerals and vitamins along with omega-3 fatty acids. They also aid in sexual health, and they may have anti-cancer properties. They are very low in carbs and calories, so they also aid in weight loss.

Crab

Crab has very little fat, is low in calories, and tastes great. It is free of carbohydrates and aids in building muscle while losing weight. It is considered healthy for the diet of expectant mothers and is a good source of riboflavin and selenium.

Mackerel

Mackerel is an oily fish that is rich in omega-3 fatty acids, helping to reduce inflammation and the risk of cardiovascular diseases, cancer and arthritis. It is also a good source of lean protein. The calcium in it also aids in burning fat and maintaining bone health.

Oyster

Oysters are aphrodisiacs and are good for sexual health. They are very low in calories, fats and carbohydrates. They are a great source of protein and keep you satiated after a meal. They are also a good source of vitamin A, vitamin E and minerals like iron, calcium and selenium.

Salmon

Salmon is one of the best sources of omega-3 fatty acids and protein in the diet. It also contains the antioxidant astaxanthin, which benefits your health. It is very dense in nutrients and promotes heart health.

Shrimp

Shrimp provides protein, selenium and niacin. They are low in calories and help in weight loss. They promote bone strength, mental health and cardiovascular health. They are also good for the eyes.

Sea Bass
Sea bass is a great source of protein and selenium and is very low in calories. The high level of omega-3 fatty acids makes it healthy, especially aiding in eye health. It is also a source of vitamin B12 and vitamin B6.

Flounder
Flounder is a heart-healthy ingredient in your diet and provides many essential nutrients.

Tilapia
Tilapia contains very little fat or calories and aids in weight loss. It also protects the body from symptoms of aging, reduces cholesterol and triglycerides and contains no carbohydrates.

Yellowtail
Yellowtail is a delicacy that is rich and fatty and a great source of omega-3 fatty acids. It is said to help in the treatment of depression and lifts the mood. It also aids in lowering blood pressure and reducing inflammation during arthritis.

Squid
It contains vitamins and minerals like vitamin B12, iron, copper and potassium. It promotes healthy blood cells and boosts the immune system. It can also aid in reducing levels of bad cholesterol or LDL.

Sardines

Sardines are good for the heart and a great source of vitamin B12. The mercury content is also minimal, and they are also high in vitamin D.

Beef
They are a great source of niacin, riboflavin and vitamin B6. The protein from beef helps to build bone strength and muscle growth. The selenium in beef supports the immune system.

Chicken
Chicken is a good source of low-fat protein, and it contributes to muscle growth and development. It is also a good source of vitamin B6, niacin and selenium. The chicken breast is considered useful in controlling homocysteine levels, which helps to reduce the risk of heart diseases.

Duck
The monounsaturated fat found in duck helps to reduce LDL and increasing HDL. It is a good source of niacin, riboflavin, thiamine, zinc and iron. It supports cardiovascular health and is also rich in vitamin B6.

Goat
The vitamin B in goat meat helps to burn fat in the body. It contains a lot of lean protein and very little saturated fat, which aids in weight loss. The selenium and choline content of this meat help to prevent cancer. It is leaner than meat from beef, pork or chicken.

Lamb

Lamb is a good source of protein that is of high quality and contains vitamins and minerals. The nutrients of this meat promote growth and development of muscles. It is also helpful in maintaining healthy levels of cholesterol and is a good source of selenium.

Guinea Fowl

Guinea fowl has low levels of cholesterol and fats and is a healthy choice for your meal. The eggs are also healthy and contain vitamin E, vitamin D3 and vitamin A. The meat of the fowl supports heart health and boosts mental health.

Another great source of high-quality protein is eggs. They are a very common part of the Mediterranean diet and are especially good for people who don't consume any meat. You can opt for chicken eggs, duck eggs or even quail eggs.

Chapter 9:
Keto-Mediterranean Fruits and Dairy Products

Fruits are healthy foods that should be part of your diet, consumed whole and fresh in order to obtain the maximum nutritional benefit from them. However, processed fruit juices are not as beneficial since they are filled with added sugar and preservatives. Unlike vegetables, however, you will need to control your fruit portions due to the higher content of carbohydrates. As mentioned earlier, fruits like mangoes and bananas are rich in natural sugar and should be limited.

Some of the recommended Keto-Mediterranean fruit are listed below along with their health benefits:

Apple
Apples contain flavonoids, which are antioxidants that can help to reduce the risk of diabetes and asthma. They can also help cleanse the oral cavity. The skin of the apple should not be peeled since it contains most of the vitamins.

Apricot

Apricots are a great source of Vitamin A, which promotes eye health. They provide iron to fight anemia and have pectin, which treats constipation. They are diet-friendly and benefit the skin and bone health. For pregnant women, apricots are considered helpful and nutritious.

Cherry

Cherries are a popular fruit of many varieties. The sour variety contains a better nutritional profile compared to the sweeter cherries. They contain vitamin A, vitamin C, potassium, copper and manganese.

Dates

Dates are very nutritious and high in fiber content. They contain antioxidants, help to promote brain health and are also a great natural sweetener. The fruit can also aid in natural labor. They also contain various vitamins and minerals.

Grapes

Grapes are packed with vitamin C and vitamin K. and antioxidants, which can protect against chronic disease. Resveratrol in grapes is a key nutrient that can benefit your body. Grapes can also decrease levels of blood sugar in the body and protect from Type 2 Diabetes.

Cucumbers

Cucumber is a fruit. It is low in calories and has large amounts of water and dietary fiber, aiding in weight loss and increasing hydration.

Melon
Melons contain heart-supporting elements like vitamin C, fiber, potassium and choline. The potassium helps to reduce blood pressure.

Olives
Olives have great antioxidant properties that reduce the risk of heart diseases, cancer, and return blood cholesterol and blood pressure to a normal level. Olives are also said to benefit bone health and boost iron intake in the body.

Orange
A single orange can provide you with a variety of vitamins and minerals. It is a rich source of vitamin C and can significantly reduce the risk of ischemic stroke in women. It also helps to prevent damage to skin and lowers bad cholesterol or high blood sugar.

Pomegranate
This fruit is very rich in vitamin C and potassium. It is also a good source of fiber. This fruit helps in digestion and protection against heart disease, arthritis and Alzheimer's.

Strawberry
Strawberries are a very rich source of antioxidants and protect against free radicals. It is good for weight management and helps to reduce blood sugar regulation. This fruit also has anti-microbial properties and is good for the heart and immune system.

Clementine

Clementine's are rich in nutrients that are vital for health. They contain a lot of calcium, potassium, phosphorus and magnesium. They provide vitamin C and folate. Clementine's promote good vision and is beneficial for the skin and digestive system.

Blueberry

Blueberries are quite low in carbohydrates and are rich in polyphenols that are good for health. They also contain vitamin C, vitamin E, vitamin B6, vitamin K and manganese.

Blackberry

They are a good source of vitamin C and contain a relatively low amount of sugar compared to other fruit. They also provide manganese, vitamin K and vitamin E.

Peach

Peaches contain nutrients and vitamins like vitamin E, vitamin A and vitamin C. Peaches are low in calories and boost metabolism. The catechins in peaches help to burn calories and aid in weight loss.

Fig

This fruit is rich in fiber, and this keeps you full for a long time. It also aids in relieving constipation. Figs are a good source of vitamin A, vitamin B1 and vitamin B2. They can also aid in lowering blood sugar and blood cholesterol levels. The calcium content of a fig helps to prevent osteoporosis.

Avocados

They are a good source of Vitamin E and folate. Avocados contain monounsaturated fats that aid in lowering bad cholesterol levels. The cold-pressed oil obtained from this fruit is nearly as healthy as olive oil. It is also a very versatile fruit and can be used in many different dishes.

Tangerine

They provide a lot of nutrients like potassium and thiamine to the body. They are a low-calorie fruit that contain more vitamin A than almost any other fruit. The high content of fiber relieves constipation, and it also aids in iron absorption.

Tomato

Tomatoes are not native to the Mediterranean but are always found in Mediterranean kitchens. They are packed with lycopene, which is an antioxidant that protects the heart. They also contain a lot of vitamin C and add flavor to all kinds of dishes.

Pear

This fruit is full of fiber and is beneficial for skin health. It is also beneficial in treating diverticulosis and aids in preventing cardiovascular diseases. Pears are a detoxifying fruit and aid in digestion. They are a good source of vitamin C.

The following are some of the dairy products that will benefit your Ketogenic Mediterranean diet process and help you stay healthy while losing weight.

Brie

The protein found in Brie can provide your body with every amino acid it requires. This cheese has lower fat and calorie content than other cheeses. It is also lower in carbohydrate content. Every ounce of Brie has about 6 grams of protein and 8 grams of fat.

Feta

Feta cheese is usually made with milk from sheep or goats. It has a good amount of vitamin B and calcium. It also has bacteria that are beneficial for gut health. Due to the high saturated fat and sodium content, you should consume this cheese carefully. It is considered one of the best cheeses in a diet meant for weight loss.

Chevre

Chevre is a goat milk cheese that provides healthy fats to the body. It also provides probiotic bacteria and is easier to digest than some other cheeses. It aids in reducing hunger cravings and is a good source of calcium and protein.

Haloumi

It is considered a healthy cheese that is very low in carbohydrate content. It is naturally salty and is a good option for the vegetarian diet.

Pecorino

It is a good source of calcium, potassium and protein. It is usually used as an alternative for Parmesan cheese and has a sharper taste, so a little is usually enough.

Yogurt

Yogurts are usually high in protein, calcium, probiotics and vitamins. They aid in maintaining bone health and can protect from osteoporosis. Yogurt aids in the digestive process and is a good source of protein in a diet meant for weight loss.

Ricotta

Ricotta cheese has a texture that is like cottage cheese, although it is lighter. It can provide a lot of calcium and protein in even a small amount. This cheese is low in sodium content and higher in phosphorous and vitamin content. It is also a good source of omega fatty acids.

Manchego

This cheese is commonly consumed in Spain, is a very good source of protein and can be eaten even if you have high cholesterol. It provides a lot of calcium, which ensures good bone health and is recommended for pregnant women, children and the elderly. It is also a lactose-free cheese and works as a laxative too.

The following are the best oils for the Keto-Mediterranean diet:

Olive Oil

When it comes to oils, your best bet is olive oil. We have already mentioned in previous chapters how this oil is beneficial to your health. Olives or olive oil is quite central to the diet of the Mediterranean region. You can opt to have whole olives in your diet or use the oil for cooking or flavoring your food. Olive oil is the main dietary fat source that is used in cooking and baking or in dressings on salads and vegetables. The highest amount of health-promoting fats can be found in extra virgin olive oil, which will also provide you with a lot of phytonutrients and many other micronutrients that are important for your body.

Avocado oil

It is very rich in oleic acid that is a healthy fat. It helps to reduce bad cholesterol and aids in improving heart health. This oil has a high amount of lutein that is an antioxidant that benefits eye health. It also enhances nutrient absorption in the body and can improve the skin. It can also help to reduce symptoms of arthritis and gum disease.

Canola Oil

Canola oil is a healthy cooking oil that contains omega-3 fatty acids as well as omega 6 fatty acids. The reduced saturated fat in this oil helps to reduce cholesterol. It is also rich in vitamin E and vitamin K, which aid in maintaining healthy skin and reducing signs of aging like wrinkles and blemishes.

Anti-Inflammatory Keto (30% More Effective)

From all the information given above, you can understand why we recommend these food items and ingredients in your diet. They are all keto-friendly, and are already a part of the Mediterranean diet, aiding in overall wellbeing while helping you to

Chapter 10:
Finding Your Carb Sweet Spot

The Ketogenic Mediterranean diet is a very low carb diet but not one that eliminates carbohydrates. In the limited quantity of carbohydrates that are allowed in the diet, it is important to consider what you should eat. To enjoy the best benefits of this diet, you should include carbs that will still let your body stay in the state of ketosis to keep burning fats successfully. For this, you must find a way to benefit from the carbohydrates in your diet without suffering any of the negative impacts.

Carbohydrates have their benefits. They help to increase leptin levels, improve libido, increase metabolism and increase anabolism; however, we rarely reap these benefits because it is easy to consume too many carbohydrates and then you are just impacted by the negative aspect. Eating too much carbohydrate loaded food and at the wrong time will only lead to excessive body weight. If you completely cut them off, then you will miss out on the performance-enhancing benefit of carbs. So, the question is how to find the carb sweet spot while maintaining ketosis in the Ketogenic Mediterranean diet.

The carbohydrate-limiting factor can be confusing. You might be wondering what you can or cannot eat in the form of carbs and how can you eat carbs without affecting ketosis in your body. If you follow the Mediterranean food guide while on the keto diet, you don't really have to worry about the bad carb or good carb options. Most of your food will be healthy on this diet anyway. Occasionally eating a little bit of a bad carb might work as a treat for you too.

In the ketogenic diet, it is recommended to eat complex carbohydrate foods and avoid simple carbohydrates. Complex carbohydrates include unrefined whole grain bread, unrefined brown rice, beans, chickpeas, carrots and leafy greens. Simple carbohydrates include white bread, white rice, processed cereals and refined pasta, candy, and fruit juices. You should limit the low carb foods to sources such as berries and leafy greens, which will allow you to stay in the limit of daily carb consumption while getting enough fiber and micronutrients. You need to kick off the habit of consuming refined grains, sugar and such simple carbohydrates that will compromise the process of ketosis.

The best options that will help you stay healthy are complex carbohydrate sources like eggplant, broccoli, and asparagus. Potatoes are a bad carb that you need to avoid since a single large potato will cross your daily carb limit quite easily. When you are on a keto diet, you should stick to unrefined complex carbs that will help to lower your blood glucose levels. This way you won't have to depend on any glucose supporting supplements.

The complex carbs will provide enough energy to keep your body functioning and healthy. The sources we recommended in this diet will also support a healthy gut and provide you with essential micronutrients.

To determine how much carbohydrate the body will need without gaining weight, you must keep a few factors in mind.

Your body type plays a role in determining its own ability to handle any carbohydrates. Ectomorphs are more capable of consuming carbs than their counterparts. Thus, the former should consume more compared to the latter.

The body fat to muscle ratio in a person will help to determine how tolerant his or her body is with carbs. People who have higher muscle mass and lesser body fat are more tolerant and can consume more carbohydrates. Those with higher fats and less muscle tend to store fat and should consume fewer carbohydrates.

The amount of carbs a person requires also depends on their activity levels. The more energy they burn, the more carbs they need. The more sedentary their lifestyle, the fewer carbs they require.

Anti-Inflammatory Keto (30% More Effective)

These factors will give you an idea about how many carbs you should consume in your diet, and you can adjust the numbers accordingly. Ultimately you must remember that the Ketogenic Mediterranean diet is very low in carbohydrates and only requires the minimum essential amount of this macronutrient.

Some dietitians also recommend that the individual increase their awareness of what the body needs. If you feel that you had a high-performance day and your body needs a little extra carbohydrate, then it is okay to provide it with the carbs in moderation. If you feel that you had a very sedentary day with barely any physical activity, then you probably don't require any at all.

On days that you skip your regular workout, you can also afford to skip your carbohydrate dose. Your body is the best guide that you should listen to. Listen to common sense and fight any unhealthy cravings at the beginning of your diet and later you should listen to your body and eat accordingly. For instance, some people find it healthier to eat three meals in one day while others eat smaller portions throughout the day. It can differ from person to person, and there is no single right or wrong way. It takes time to develop body awareness and can be very easy to mix up signals sent by the body. Take the time to learn and get to recognize its needs.

In the ketogenic diet, the usual carb limit is total carbs of 35 grams and net carbs of 25 grams; however, there is no specific number that the Ketogenic Mediterranean diet recommends. You shouldn't punish yourself for consuming some fruit in the evening. Each person has a different carb limit that they should set. This limit can differ from person to person, and even for that individual, it can be different on any given day.

Achieving ketosis will depend on many other factors and not just the carbohydrate intake of that day. There are people whose bodies kick into ketosis only when carbs are below 35 grams while others can consume more and still burn fat. This can make it challenging to determine what your limit is. Until you figure it out, you can use the general ketogenic diet limit for carbs that we mentioned earlier. It is found to be effective for most people who started on this diet and should work for you too. A lot of people also found that reducing the carbs to 20 grams helps to speed up ketosis in the body. It can help to maintain constant ketosis and losing weight.

The following are carbohydrate sources that you should and should not eat to maintain ketosis:

- Don't eat wheat, rice, corn or any such grains that are loaded with carbs.
- Avoid honey, maple syrup and other such sugar sources.
- Avoid fruits like bananas that are rich in sugar carbs.
- Don't eat potatoes and yams.

Anti-Inflammatory Keto (30% More Effective)

- Eat a moderate quantity of berries because they contain fewer carbs than other fruit and are also a powerhouse of antioxidants.
- Add avocados to your diet, as they are low in carbs, high in fat and fiber and are great for keto.
- Eat more lean meats like poultry and fish.
- Eat leafy greens that have a very little digestible fat and mostly contain fiber and water.
- Eat high-fat dairy like hard cheeses and fatty creams.
- Eat macadamia nuts, walnut and sunflower seeds. They are low in carbs but high in fiber and fat.
- Use coconut oil, avocado oil and canola oil.

You must understand that everyone has a different carb sweet spot for ketosis. We have given you the general limit for carbs in your diet, but it may not work for certain people and it might stop working at a certain point in your diet as well. If this happens, you should consider some other factors that will then contribute to determining the limit and your ketosis.

The process of keto-adaptation changes your body's ketone burning ability and your carb limit. Every person's body can burn ketones for energy. During keto-adaptation, mitochondria in the body starts working more efficiently and replicates. They then provide other cells with the ability to burn ketones for fuel instead of using sugar. This kind of adaptation helps the body to enter ketosis quickly. The more adapted you get to the ketogenic diet, the more carbs you can consume while maintaining ketosis over time.

If you want to take advantage of this adaptation, you should maintain the diet strictly for at least four to six months. During this period don't make any changes to the given plan and follow it blindly. You shouldn't increase your carbohydrate intake from 35 grams during the keto-adaptation period so that there is constant ketosis and your cells get used to the process. It is the only way you can reap the adaptation benefits later.

Another factor that is important to boost ketosis is exercise. A lot of people try to avoid this aspect and so they don't reap the total benefits of the ketogenic diet. It is for this reason that we said that adapting to the Mediterranean lifestyle would help to reap more benefit from the ketogenic diet too.

The people of that region are quite proactive in exercising and maintaining fitness and thus have a lower incidence of obesity. If you start the right type of exercise, it can help you to achieve ketosis even faster and boost the level of ketones in your body. If you want a rapid onset of ketosis, you should give serious consideration to high-intensity training. It will aid in depleting the stored glycogen in your body. Low-intensity training can be used to encourage more fat-burning.

When you are beginning the Ketogenic Mediterranean diet, focus first on depleting the storage of glycogen. This will push the body into ketosis faster. You can do this by practicing an hour of some high-intensity exercise in the morning like heavyweights, cross fit, and HIIT. When the workout is complete, you should give your body time to recover. Make sure you rehydrate and take some mineral supplements. Also, avoid eating anything till mealtime.

When the glycogen level in your body is depleted, low-intensity training will help to increase ketones and burning fat. This can be done by about half an hour of brisk walking or cycling before breakfast. If you do all this at the right time every day, it will help you achieve ketosis quite quickly. You will also be able to increase the carbohydrate limit in your diet without compromising on your ketone levels. You should also remember not to over-do high-intensity exercise as it can overwhelm your body and impair the ketosis ability of your body.

Stress is another important factor to consider since it can impair the ability of your body to carry out ketosis and will decrease your carbohydrate intake limit in the diet. The stress hormone levels increase in people who suffer from anxiety or stress on a regular basis. Cortisol is one of the stress hormones released during stress, and it increases gluconeogenesis in the body, which in turn decreases insulin sensitivity in the body. This results in increased blood sugar for a longer period, and thus the body does not require ketone production. You must remember that cortisol is not the enemy since it is a hormone that helps in different situations. There will be an issue if your body is incapable of producing cortisol.

The problem is stress in the process of ketosis and your diet. There are certain stressors that you need to avoid like worrying about the future or overwhelming yourself with work. A lot of people get stressed by thinking too much about past mistakes instead of moving on. Eating too little or exercising too much will also stress your body and mind. It is important to pace yourself, rest and give your body time to recover. This way you can avoid stress and alleviate the levels of stress hormones that limit the body's ketone production abilities. Stress will prevent you from losing weight and affect your ability to maintain muscle mass too. You need to avoid all such factors while you are on the Ketogenic Mediterranean diet if you want to see real results and stay healthy. Certain strategies will help you reduce stress and maintain ketosis. This includes eating the right quantity of calories in your diet, avoiding excessive exercise, improving the sleep cycle and practicing meditation. Meditation is considered very helpful in reducing stress and decreasing cortisol levels in the body.

Protein intake is also a factor that can block ketosis in your body. If your diet consists of too much protein, it floods the body with amino acids. In response to this, insulin will be released, and the body gets the signal that enough energy is available in the form of the amino acids. Due to this, they don't kickstart the process of ketosis and fat burning for energy. Thus, you can see that high protein meals can prevent ketosis in the body or cause a stall at some point. You shouldn't just focus on restricting carbohydrates during your diet but also on maintaining the right level of all the macros. The right balance in your diet will make a big difference.

The 35-gram total carb limit is generally ideal for everyone at least in the first few months of the ketogenic diet. It is important to consider the factors we mentioned like your stress level, exercise, and protein intake. They will all help in determining if your carb limit should be reduced or increased to improve the process of ketosis in your body. Finding your carb limit can be more complex than you might expect so try not to experiment too much in the beginning.

When you want to find your carb limit, certain steps will help. Keep track of your ketones with the help of a blood ketone meter. Increase your intake of carbs and keep tracking the ketone levels over time. First, give your body time to establish ketosis for some time by using the 35-gram limit. Then, after a while, increase your limit by 5 grams each day. These carbs should still be healthy for you and not some candies or simple sugars. Such simple carbs will rapidly increase your insulin levels and kick you out of ketosis. Increasing complex carbs from plant-based sources will help. Take the ketone measurement in your blood at the same time every single day. This will help you in seeing if the increased carbohydrates decreased your blood ketone level.

After increasing the limit, if you see that the ketone level has not decreased, you can increase the limit a little more after time. Repeat the tracking process again and decrease the carb limit of you see that the ketone level decrease. You should always aim to maintain a level of ketosis according to the weight goal that you have set. For those who want to lose significant weight, it should be in a state of deep ketosis with 1.5 mmol/L to 3.0 mmol/L. Blood ketone meters are the only way to determine the level of ketosis accurately. During the first couple of days of the ketogenic diet, most people will find that they are in a state of light ketosis. Deep ketosis kicks in only after a couple of weeks. The tips in this chapter aim to help you kick in ketosis even more rapidly. While you are maintaining the limit of 35 grams of carbs, monitor your progress. If it is working well and helping you lose enough weight, there is no reason to increase or decrease your limit until you reach your goal or hit a weight stall. Experimenting too much for no reason will only complicate the process for you.

Your carb limit will depend on factors like sleep and activity that we discussed earlier. If you are exercising a little extra today, you can add a few extra grams of carbohydrate for that day without guilt. It takes time, patience and persistence to find the carb limit for ketosis in your body. You must track the changes in your body and life to get the best results while you follow the Ketogenic Mediterranean diet.

For athletes or high-intensity trainers, carbohydrates can play a major role. They cannot always afford to consume too few carbs in their diet. For beginners in high-intensity training, the targeted ketogenic version of the diet is recommended. In this case, the person can consume an extra 10-20 grams of carbs that are easily digestible. This should be done about half an hour before they exercise. This is only for beginners and not for athletes and regular trainers. These people might require the cyclical version of the ketogenic diet. This version involves a couple of days of increased carb followed by the ketogenic regime the rest of the week. It helps combine ketosis with carbohydrates for improving the athlete's strength and performance. They need to deplete their glycogen stores before they start the refeeding cycle.

Ketone boosting supplements are another factor that you can consider for boosting ketosis in your body. One is ketone salt, which is a powder containing ketone bodies with minerals. Usually, they contain calcium, potassium, magnesium or sodium and these are bound with acetoacetate or beta-hydroxybutyrate.

Consumption of ketone salts helps to significantly increase ketone levels without the waiting period required in the standard diet. But there are studies that show that these ketone salts can impair the body's ability to maintaining ketosis in the long term. The salts should not be used as a replacement for the limit of carbs either.

The standard ketogenic diet is much more beneficial in the long run and is a healthier option too. You can consider certain ketone salts if you suffer from some mineral deficiency that it can act as a supplement for. MCT oil is the other supplement used in ketosis. MCT stands for medium chain triglycerides, and these can be broken down in the liver to ketone bodies. This happens whether the body has entered ketosis. They are saturated fats unlike any other type of saturated fat. They will help to skip the part of fat digestion and are directly converted into ketone bodies in the liver regardless of following the ketogenic diet.

In natural form, these are found in coconuts, but the easiest way is to take them in the form of the MCT oil supplement. The best supplement is one that contains caprylic acid. This MCT is known to get digested and converted to ketones faster than other types. You must remember that none of the ketone boosting supplements will benefit you like the actual ketogenic diet and they should only be used as a last resort or temporarily.

Everyone will not get the same result from the same carb limit. The ketone levels in your body will depend on the level of activity you perform, the amount of protein you consume, your stress levels and your keto-adaptation period. For this reason, some people thrive on a higher intake of carbohydrates while others require less. Supplements will help you to a certain extent, but the Ketogenic Mediterranean diet is your best bet for a healthy process of weight loss. As you keep reading, you will also learn about how intermittent fasting will aid this process.

Anti-Inflammatory Keto (30% More Effective)

Chapter 11:
Intermittent Fasting

The intermittent fasting diet is one of the most popular fitness and health trends in the world. People use this method to improve their health, change their lifestyles and lose weight. Many studies talk about the powerful effects that this lifestyle has on a person's brain and body. Some studies also show that this lifestyle can help you live a longer life. We will cover some of the basics of intermittent fasting in this chapter.

Intermittent fasting is an eating pattern where you shift between periods of eating and fasting. This pattern does not specify which food you should eat but tells you when you should be consuming those foods. Therefore, one cannot use the conventional term "diet" to describe this eating. As mentioned earlier, this is an eating pattern. Some methods of intermittent fasting involve a sixteen-hour fast or a 24-hour fast at least twice a week.

Throughout human evolution, human beings have practiced fasting. Our ancestors did not have refrigerators, grocery stores or food available throughout the year. There were times when they did not find any food that they could eat. As a result, human beings could survive and function without any food for a long period. Fasting is considered more natural when compared to consuming at least four meals a day. Some people also fast for spiritual or religious reasons, and many religions like Islam, Hinduism, Judaism, Christianity and Buddhism promote fasting.

Intermittent Fasting Methods

You can follow different eating patterns if you choose to follow the intermittent fasting lifestyle. Each of these patterns will involve splitting the week or day into fasting and eating periods. You either eat nothing or very little during the fasting period. The most popular methods of intermittent fasting are:

Eat-Stop-Eat

In this method, you will need to fast for at least twenty-four hours either once or twice a week. For example, you could skip dinner tonight and not eat any food until dinner the following night.

The 16/8 Method

The 16/8 method, also known as the Lean Gains protocol, requires you to skip breakfast every day and restrict the eating period to eight hours only. You can eat between 1 PM and 9 PM or any other period depending on your convenience. You will then need to fast for sixteen hours.

The 5:2 Diet

In this method, you will normally eat on five days of the week but consume only 600 calories on two non-consecutive days.

These methods will help you lose weight, if you do not consume more calories than needed during the eating period. People prefer the 16/8 method since that is the easiest method to stick to, and it is sustainable.

Alternate Day Fasting
As the name suggests, in this fasting you only fast on alternate days. There are variations of this method. In some of the variations, you can consume 500 calories on alternate days while on others you are asked to follow a strict fast and only drink water. The benefits of this diet are the same as those of any other type of intermittent fasting. A strict diet can be overwhelming for a beginner, so you can modify this diet to suit your needs. However, you should be prepared to overcome pangs of hunger on some days.

Skipping Meals Spontaneously
As the name suggests, there is no plan for this diet. You can reap the benefits of the intermittent fasting diet without having to plan elaborate meals. This is a simple variation to follow since you only need to skip meals occasionally. When you are not hungry or are occupied with some work, you can skip a meal since you will not be thinking about food. People do not have to eat every two hours, and your body will not starve if you do not give it food every two hours. The human

body has been designed in a way to help you go without food for a long period. It is all right to miss two meals occasionally since it gives your body the opportunity to remove any toxins. So, if you are not hungry, you can skip the meal.

Every variation of intermittent fasting is effective, and it would be best for you to choose a variation that works best for you.

How Does Intermittent Fasting Affect Your Cells and Hormones?

Your body goes through several changes at the molecular and cellular levels when you fast. For instance, your body will adjust to all the hormone levels and make use of the stored fat in the body to produce energy. Your cells will also begin to repair and alter your genes. Let us look at some changes that will occur in your body when you fast.

Human Growth Hormone

The growth hormone levels will skyrocket. This helps you lose weight, shed fat and gain muscle mass.

Insulin

The levels of insulin in your blood will drop rapidly, and your body's sensitivity to insulin will improve. Your body can access the stored body fat easily if the levels of insulin are low.

Cellular Repair

When your body is in the fasting state, your cells will begin the repair process. This means that the cells will remove or digest dysfunctional and old proteins that develop in the cells. This process is called autophagy.

Gene Expression

Intermittent fasting will lead to some changes in the functions of genes that are associated with your immunity and longevity.

These changes in cell function, gene expression and hormone levels are the factors responsible for the health benefits of this eating pattern.

A Powerful Weight Loss Tool

Most people choose the intermittent fasting eating pattern to lose weight. When you reduce the number of meals you consume every day, you will automatically reduce your caloric intake. As mentioned earlier, the changes in the hormones aid in weight loss. In addition to this, intermittent fasting also helps to increase the quantity of noradrenaline or norepinephrine, the fat-burning hormone.

Your metabolic rate may increase between 3.6-14% because of the changes in your hormones. Since you will consume fewer calories and burn more calories, you will lose weight since the calorie equation will change.

Many studies show that intermittent fasting is an easy way to lose weight. A study showed that this eating pattern would help a person lose at least 3-8% of their weight in 24 weeks. This is a significant amount of loss, which is more than any other weight loss method. In the same study, people also lost at least 7% of their waist circumference which indicates that intermittent fasting helps to burn belly fat which accumulates around your organs and leads to numerous diseases. You should, however, keep in mind that intermittent fasting is successful since it ensures that you consume fewer calories. If you binge or eat large quantities of food during your eating periods, you will not lose any weight.

Health Benefits

There are many studies conducted on intermittent fasting using both animals and human beings as subjects. These studies show that intermittent fasting helps to improve the health of your brain and body, and aid in weight loss. Let us look at some of the benefits of intermittent fasting.

Weight Loss

As mentioned earlier, intermittent fasting will help you lose belly fat and weight, and you don't have to restrict your caloric intake consciously.

Insulin Resistance

Through intermittent fasting, one can overcome insulin resistance. This helps to reduce the level of blood sugar by at least 6%. This will protect your body against Type 2 Diabetes.

Inflammation
Studies show that intermittent fasting reduces the symptoms of inflammation, thereby reducing the risk of developing numerous chronic diseases.

Heart Health
Intermittent fasting will reduce bad cholesterol, blood sugar, inflammatory markers, insulin resistance and blood triglycerides, thereby reducing the probability of developing heart diseases.

Cancer
Many animal studies suggest that the intermittent fasting eating pattern helps to prevent the growth of cancerous cells.

Brain Health
The brain hormone, BDNF, is released in large quantities when you follow the intermittent fasting diet. This hormone will aid in the growth of new cells in the brain and may prevent the development of Alzheimer's.

Anti-Aging
Studies conducted on rats showed that intermittent fasting extends lifespan. This study showed that rats that were fasting lived at least 36-83% longer than rats that did not fast.

You should keep in mind that further research must be conducted to understand the benefits of intermittent fasting. The studies that have been conducted were short-term, small or conducted on animals. Some questions about how intermittent fasting affects human beings still need to be answered.

Makes Your Lifestyle Simpler

It is simple to eat healthy, but it is hard to maintain it. The main obstacle is the work you will need to put in to cooking healthy meals. You will need to plan your meals and procure your ingredients in advance. Intermittent fasting will make things easier since you do not have too many dishes to cook since you will be consuming fewer meals overall. You will also have fewer dishes to clean. It is for this reason that people who look for life-hacks follow the intermittent fasting diet. This diet will simplify your life and improve your health.

Who Should Avoid or Be Careful?

Not everyone can follow intermittent fasting or adopt this eating pattern as their lifestyle. If you are underweight or have an eating disorder, you should speak to your physician before you adopt this eating pattern. In some cases, this eating pattern is downright harmful.

Should Women Fast?

Some studies state that intermittent fasting is not as beneficial for women when compared to men. For instance, a study showed that intermittent fasting helped to improve insulin sensitivity in men and worsened the control of blood sugar in women.

According to some studies, intermittent fasting is not as beneficial for women when compared to men. Human studies are currently unavailable on this topic, and most studies have been conducted on rats. Studies showed that intermittent fasting could lead to infertility or missed menstrual cycles in female rats.

Some women reported that their menstrual period stopped when they adopted the intermittent fasting eating pattern. The menstrual cycle went back to normal when they began to eat normally. It is for this reason that women should be extremely careful when they adopt the intermittent fasting eating method. Women should follow a separate guideline, and ease into the practice slowly. They should stop immediately if they have any issues with menstruation. If you have any issues with fertility or are trying to conceive, you should avoid this eating pattern.

Side Effects and Safety

One of the main side effects of intermittent fasting is hunger. You will also feel weak until your body can handle the decreased quantity of glucose. There is a possibility that your brain may not perform as well as it used to until it adapts. As mentioned earlier, this is only temporary since it will take your body some time to adapt to the new schedule.

Anti-Inflammatory Keto (30% More Effective)

If you suffer from any medical conditions, you should check with your physician before you follow this eating pattern. This is especially important if you:

- Have trouble with the regulation of blood sugar
- Have diabetes
- Are on certain medications
- Have suffered from eating disorders in the past
- Have low blood pressure
- Are underweight
- Are pregnant or breastfeeding
- Are a woman who has a history of amenorrhea
- Are a woman who is trying to conceive

There is nothing dangerous about intermittent fasting since your body will come to no harm if you do not eat for a while. This is the case if you are well nourished and healthy.

Chapter 12:
The Mediterranean Ketogenic Diet

Nutritionists and doctors have conducted numerous scientific studies over the last decade, which has encouraged them to revise their idea of what a healthy diet is. Studies have helped people learn more about the mechanisms and the causes of cancer, arteriosclerosis and diabetes. It is for this reason that the idea of a healthy food pyramid is now disregarded. Grains, beans, starchy vegetables and bread are no longer used as the basis for any diet.

New scientific data and research prove that healthy fat is of utmost importance in a diet. Nutritionists are now combining these principles with the Mediterranean diet. This diet includes a healthy amount of fresh vegetables and nuts and is called the Ketogenic Mediterranean diet. The traditional Mediterranean diet allows you to consume fruit, vegetables, potatoes and nuts, whole grains and olive oil. You can also consume moderate amounts of lean meat, poultry, fish, eggs, dairy products and moderate quantities of red wine. The emphasis is only placed on the consumption of whole and fresh foods, and to minimize the consumption of processed and packaged food.

Anti-Inflammatory Keto (30% More Effective)

In a traditional ketogenic diet, at least fifty percent of your food intake should come from fat like butter, coconut oil, eggs, raw nuts, avocado, poultry, red meats, cheese, fish and shellfish. This diet does not include sugar, whole grains, starchy vegetables, beans and flour. We talked about ketosis in the first few chapters of the book. Ketosis is a metabolic state in which your body will break down the stored fat to produce energy. Your body shifts into this state since there are no carbohydrates that it can use to produce energy. This breakdown will lead to the formation of ketone bodies that are used by your body as energy. For you to reach the state of ketosis, you should only consume fifty grams of carbohydrates a day. This means that you can only consume 200 calories worth of carbohydrates every day. The average American consumes close to 600 calories a day, which cannot lead to fat burning.

The Mediterranean ketogenic diet uses a generous amount of coconut oil, olive oil, avocado oil, green vegetables, salads, moderate red wine, fish as the primary protein, fowl, eggs, lean meat and cheese. If you follow this diet, you must eliminate legumes, whole grains, food containing sugar and flour and starchy vegetables like corn, peas and potatoes. Fruit is a healthy choice for a snack, but it is not included in the list. You must choose the fruit with the least amount of sugar in it. This diet is different from other low-carb and ketogenic diets since it focuses more on fish, olive oil, healthy fat choices and red wine.

Studies show that the Mediterranean ketogenic diet aids in appetite reduction and weight loss. This evidence also suggests that the ketogenic diet is the most appropriate diet for people who suffer from heart disease, epilepsy and diabetes. There is some evidence that suggests that the ketogenic diet helps to reduce the growth of cancerous cells and reduces the effects of Alzheimer and Parkinson's. Apart from this, the ketogenic diet can help patients with headaches, acne, neurotrauma, sleep disorders, multiple sclerosis and autism. Some studies also show that the Ketogenic Mediterranean diet helps to reduce the glucose levels in the body during fasting periods thereby preventing insulin resistance. There is evidence that proves that this diet will help to decrease the levels of triglycerides, LD cholesterol and total cholesterol in the body.

You should remember that there is no single diet, which is good for a person because everybody is unique. You might have digestive issues, allergies or sensitivities that will require you to follow a different type of diet. People suffering from gall bladder disease cannot follow a high-fat diet. People should, however, strive to consume a diet that is rich in healthy fat; they should consume as much as fifty percent of the calories that they consume. They should also consume a moderate amount of high-quality protein, preferably freshwater fish, and lots of brightly colored and green vegetables. They should avoid the consumption of grains, flour products and starchy vegetables, and should avoid sugar, sweeteners and high fructose corn syrup. This is

Anti-Inflammatory Keto (30% More Effective)

because the sugar will increase blood sugar levels and lead to insulin resistance. This will increase the probability of developing inflammation, which leads to many degenerative diseases.

In addition to this, several nutritional supplements are anti-inflammatory and aid in controlling blood sugar. These include magnesium, omega-3 fatty acids, chromium, curcumin, lipoic acid, resveratrol and vitamin D. You can also supplement any high-fat diet with some pancreatic or digestive enzymes. You should also consume whole food fiber supplements and ensure that you choose those supplements that do not have any artificial sweeteners or sugar.

You should always ensure that you are informed when you make any decisions about your health.

Chapter 13:
Foods to Eat on IF and Sample Meal Plan

Foods to Eat

As mentioned earlier, there are no restrictions or specifications about how much food or what type of food you must consume when you follow IF, commonly known as Intermittent Fasting. You cannot expect to reap benefits from the diet if you consistently consume junk food. It is important to consume a balanced diet to maintain energy levels, lose weight and stick to the diet. If you want to follow the IF diet, you must consume food that is rich in nutrients like whole grains, fruit, vegetables, beans, nuts, lean proteins, and dairy.

Water

It is important to stay hydrated for multiple reasons, even when you are not eating. The amount of water that a person must drink depends on how active that person is. You must ensure that your urine is always pale yellow. If it is dark yellow, it means that your body is dehydrated. Dehydration can cause fatigue and lightheadedness, and if you consume very little food, you are causing extreme harm to your body.

If you do not want to drink plain water, you can add cucumber slices, lemon juice or mint leaves. This can be our little secret.

Avocado

You may wonder why you should consume avocado, a high-calorie fruit, when you are trying to lose weight. The monosaturated fat in the fruit is satiating. A study showed that it is best to consume at least half an avocado for lunch since it can keep you full for longer than if you did not consume the fruit at all.

Fish

The dietary guidelines suggest that one should consume at least eight ounces of fish every week. Fish is not only rich in protein and healthy fats but is also rich in vitamin D. If you do not consume too much food during the day, it is always a good idea to include fish in the meal since it provides enough nutrition. A lower caloric intake can affect your lucidity and cognition. It is best to include fish in your diet since it is considered brain food.

Cruciferous Vegetables

Cruciferous vegetables like Brussel sprouts, cauliflowers and broccoli are rich in fiber. When you consume food at erratic times, you must include food that is rich in fiber to improve bowel movements and prevent constipation. Fiber also helps to keep you full for a long period of time. Therefore, it is important that you consume a lot of fiber when you know you cannot eat for another 16 hours.

Potatoes

It is important to remember that not all white foods are bad for your health. Studies have concluded that potatoes are one of the most satiating foods on the planet and regular consumption of potatoes can help with weight loss. Potato chips and fries do not count.

Beans and Legumes

Beans and legumes are rich in carbohydrates that are required by the body to produce energy when you perform exercise. You should not load up on carbohydrates, but it would not hurt to add some low-calorie carbohydrates in your diet. Foods like black beans, lentils, peas and chickpeas are known to decrease body weight without restricting your caloric intake.

Probiotics

The villi in your intestines love diversity and consistency. The villi need enough nutrition, and they find it hard to survive when your body is starving or hungry, which can lead to issues like constipation. To counteract these side effects, it is important to include food that is rich in probiotics like kombucha, kraut and kefir in your diet.

Berries

Berries are often added to smoothies and are rich in vital nutrients. Strawberries are rich in vitamin C, and it is recommended that you consume one cup of strawberries at least once a week. A recent study concluded that people who consumed strawberries and blueberries regularly had a small increase in their BMI Body Mass Index over fourteen years when compared to those who did not consume berries.

Eggs

A large egg contains six grams of protein and can be cooked in a few minutes. It is important to consume as much protein as possible to build and repair muscles and tissues. A study found that people who consumed an egg instead of a bagel for breakfast ate less throughout the day and were often not as hungry.

Nuts

Nuts may be higher in calories when compared to junk food, but unlike junk food, nuts are rich in good fats. Studies have concluded that the polyunsaturated fat in walnuts can alter the physiological markers for satiety and hunger. If you are worried about your caloric intake, don't be. A study conducted in 2012 found that an ounce of almonds has 25 percent fewer calories than the number listed on the label. When you chew the almond, your teeth are unable to break the almond down completely. There is a small portion of the nut that remains intact in your body which is unabsorbed in the process of digestion.

Whole Grains

When you are on a diet, you are constantly worried about your intake of carbohydrates. You should not be worried about consuming whole grains since they are rich in protein and fiber. It is important that you consume a portion of whole grains regularly since they can boost your metabolism. Go out of your comfort zone and consume grains like bulgur, farro, kamut, freekeh, sorghum, millet, amaranth and spelt.

Sample Plan

This plan uses the 16/8 intermittent fasting pattern. If you are a beginner, you can use this meal plan to help you consume the right food at the right time. This plan will tell you what you should eat or drink and when. The plan is not detailed, and it gives you a range of options to choose from. You must ensure that you always cook your food using healthy oils and fats.

Drink (8 AM – 12 PM)

You must ensure that you drink a lot of liquid before you start to eat. If your workout in the morning, you should drink some herbal tea or a bottle of water fifteen minutes before your workout. You can also drink black coffee since it is a pre-workout booster. You should not drink too much black coffee, though. Read the last chapter to understand why.

Meal 1 (12 PM)

You should consume two eggs, either baked in coconut oil or boiled in water. Consume a bowl of spinach or any other green vegetable and a handful of mixed nuts or almonds. You should also drink two glasses of water, lime juice or herbal tea.

Meal 2 (3 PM)

You can consume 2 cups of quinoa or two sweet potatoes with 200 grams of tuna, beef or chicken. Top the potatoes with a handful of mixed nuts and green vegetables. You should drink two glasses of water with ginger and turmeric.

Meal 3 (6 PM)

You can consume 2 cups of quinoa or two sweet potatoes with 200 grams of tuna, beef or chicken. Top the potatoes with a handful of mixed nuts and green vegetables. You should drink two glasses of water with ginger and turmeric.

Meal 4 (7:45 PM)

Consume a bowl of mixed berries with one apple. Top this with sunflower seeds and cinnamon.

You can follow this sample plan for four weeks and see if it helps you. You can use this plan as a test to understand how your body responds to a change in your eating pattern. Remember that this plan is not exhaustive, and you can always shorten you're eating period. You can gradually increase the fasting period to twenty-four hours and fast for an entire day once your body is used to the intermittent fasting diet.

Chapter 14:
Fourteen: Common Mistakes

The tricky part about intermittent fasting is that there are numerous ways to do it. Generally, over time you will limit the eating window and increase the fasting window. Most people follow the 16/8 intermittent fasting pattern where they do not consume any food for sixteen hours and eat for eight hours. The different methods were covered extensively in chapter eleven. The type of intermittent fasting pattern you choose is dependent on the pattern you are comfortable with and following what best fits your lifestyle.

Since the pattern is a restrictive style of eating, you must ensure that it is safe for you to follow. If you have had eating disorders in the past, you should avoid following this diet.

Some people run into difficulties when they begin the intermittent fasting diet. They often run into those difficulties since they adopt an incorrect dietary approach. If you do choose to try intermittent fasting, you should maximize the benefits. This chapter covers some of the common mistakes that rookies make when they start the diet and helps you understand how you can avoid making those mistakes.

You Are Jumping Too Fast into Intermittent Fasting

One of the main reasons that most diets fail is that they expect you to follow a different lifestyle and steer away from your natural way of eating. This thought makes it hard for one to stick to the diet. If you are new to the intermittent fasting diet, you should never throw yourself into the twenty-four hour fast, because you will feel like hell after the fasting period. If you do want to start fasting, you should have smaller fasting periods. You can choose to fast for twelve hours and eat for twelve hours for a week, and gradually increase the fasting period. You are probably doing this already, so maybe this is the right option for you.

Binging on Junk Food

Most people are under the impression that intermittent fasting is one way to solve every health issue that they may have. It is true that intermittent fasting does help to improve your health and achieving weight loss goals. If you binge on processed food and sugar, though, this dietary regime is not going to do you any good. You must consume whole foods when you follow the intermittent fasting diet. When your body is in the fasting state, it burns the stored fat and damaged cells to produce energy, thereby helping to clean and heal the body. This implies that your body is going to be sensitive to the food you eat. If you do not nourish the body with the right nutrients, you will be hungry all the time. If you want to keep your hunger at bay, you must only consume healthy meals when you break your fast.

Restricting Calories

One of the main reasons people struggle with intermittent fasting is because they control their caloric intake during the eating period. You must learn to listen to your body and always eat until you feel full. The human body is an efficient machine and knows exactly what it needs. You should not restrict your caloric intake and consume food that is rich in fiber and fats. If you do not consume enough calories, you may starve your body.

Not Eating Enough

Some people never undo what they have done when they have fasted for hours because they worry that they will eat too much during the eating period. They believe it will be harder for them to fast during the next fasting period. If you consume fewer calories than required, you are making a huge mistake since your body will be starving. This will slow your metabolism and make it harder for you to shed fat. Regardless of whether you are restricting the quantity of food that you are eating; your body will need an enough food to ensure that the organs function. If your body is starving, you cannot function well and will not be able to think straight. If you feel weak and irritable or are finding it hard to focus, it means that you are not consuming the right number of calories. Here, you should use a food-tracking app to help you count your calories. If you want to learn more about the number of calories you need to function, you should meet a dietician or nutritionist.

Consuming the Wrong Food

When you do not eat often, you should be aware of what food you are putting into your mouth. A diet is not only about the calories, but also about the quality of food that you eat. You should always focus on your nutrition and consume food that is rich in the necessary minerals and vitamins. 500 calories of fried chips and 500 calories of avocados will digest differently and have a different effect on your metabolism and body.

You should always focus on striking a healthy balance when it comes to the macronutrients and fiber. You need to know how much to consume to ensure that your body is healthy. Experts suggest that you load half your plate with vegetables, a quarter of the plate with any lean protein (such as turkey, chicken or fish), and a quarter with healthy starch like quinoa, sweet potato, or brown rice. Since you will be eating fewer calories, ensure that the calories that you consume are nutritious and serve your body well. You should ensure that you do not consume calories from sub-par sources just because you need to consume fewer calories.

Training Harder and Eating Less

If you are not an active person and have never tried the intermittent fasting diet, you should try not to combine the two when you start dieting. You must ensure that you do not take up too much exercise when you have just started intermittent fasting. You must ease your body into fasting and train gradually. Ensure that you do not train your body too much and eat too little because this could lead to severe damage to your health. The human body does need exercise to function efficiently. You must ensure that you do not perform too much exercise since that can damage your health.

Obsessing Over the Schedule

When you follow the intermittent fasting dietary regime, you will understand your body better. You will notice the difference between hunger and cravings. You will also understand whether you are hungry since you are bored, under duress or other factors. You must remember to eat whenever you are hungry and not worry too much about the time. You can break your fast early if you want to eat. You must learn to listen to your body and understand what it needs. It is all right if you were unable to fast for 16 hours. You must ensure that you do not constantly deviate from your schedule.

Not Hydrating Enough

Most amateurs do not drink enough water. You must remember that your body needs to be hydrated to keep the hunger at bay. Water also helps remove the toxins found in your body. You must ensure that you drink at least eight glasses of water a day.

Taking it too Far

You must remember that intermittent fasting is not the best solution for everyone to maintain metabolic health, weight loss, or for increasing longevity. If you have tried the pattern and felt miserable after it, you should re-evaluate if this eating plan is right for you. Some people will tell you that your body can starve for hours and days since our ancestors' bodies did too. What they forget to mention is that this happened tens of thousands of years ago when food was not readily available. This does not mean that this is the right option for you.

Everybody is not built to sustain intermittent fasting. Traditional schools of medicine and health like Ayurveda define people differently based on their experiences with fasting. For instance, Ayurveda has divided people into three types Kapha, Vata and Pitta. The first type of person has extra fat in his body, slow metabolism and is never hungry in the mornings. This person can follow the intermittent fasting pattern with ease. The second type of individual has a varying appetite, can only handle fasting at times and will be thrown out of balance if he or she makes fasting a regular thing. The last type of individual has a strong appetite and cannot stick to intermittent fasting. If he or she does choose to fast, his or her body will be imbalanced, and this could lead to numerous issues.

If you find that intermittent fasting feels like a strain on your body and mind, you should ask yourself this question: is the eating pattern worth the change in the quality of my life?

Chapter 15: Tips and Tricks

Some of the tips in the chapter are evident, but it is difficult to stick to the diet for most people. When you keep this in mind, you will be able to stick to the diet. The tips mentioned in this chapter will help you stick to the intermittent fasting with ease.

Start Small
Intermittent fasting is not a diet, but a habit. It takes time for a habit to integrate into your life. It is for this reason that you must start slowly because your body will need time to adapt to the new style. It takes at least two months to develop a habit before it becomes an involuntary action. Additionally, if you fail to stick to the diet at times, it does not mean that you cannot develop the habit. It only means that it may take you longer to develop it as a habit.

Always Train in a Fastened State
It is always a good idea to train when the fasting period has ended since the blood sugar levels are at their lowest. This helps to burn stored fat, thereby helping you lose weight. When you perform the

exercise in the fastened state, your body will learn to deal better with glucose.

Find a Friend

When you have someone to help you while you fast and to hold you accountable, you will make more of an effort to stick to the challenge. You can establish an arrangement that works best for both of you.

Always Prepare your Meals in Advance

It is recommended that you prepare your first meal in advance and devour it when you end your fast. If the food is not ready, you might eat readily available junk food instead.

Keep Yourself Busy

You must keep yourself busy when you are fasting. If you do not have much to do, you might constantly check the clock while you wait for the fasting period to end. Alternatively, you can leave your body in the fasting state when you sleep.

Think about Food

It is all right to think about what you are going to eat when the fasting period is over. You do not have to suppress your urges since you are going to think about food constantly. You can look forward to the lovely meals you will consume immediately after the fasting period.

Stay Hydrated

As mentioned earlier, it is important to keep yourself hydrated. If you are bored of plain water, you can add some mint leaves or lemon juice to it. Ensure that you do not add sugar since it could negate the effects of fasting.

Stop Looking at Results Each Day

You must never look for results every single day. You must remember that weight loss is a long process. Instead, count every day when you have stuck to your schedule as a victory since that will bring you one step closer to achieving your goal.

Be Smart and Sensible

It is important that you pay attention to your body. Remember that it takes time for the body to adapt to intermittent fasting. If your body was okay with you fasting for twelve hours today, add an extra hour tomorrow and see what happens. You must learn your limits, but never make it too easy for yourself, or you will end up exactly where you started.

Motivate Yourself

You should ensure that every fast does not end in a feast. You must remember that fasting is about teaching and training your body to become efficient and use what you eat wisely. You must reward yourself with some good food. Never fast only for that reward since the result would then become the reward. You can pat yourself on the back or consume a big meal on a day when you do not fast, but never because you feel like it. This will create a positive association between your mind and the diet.

Some Additional Tips

In this section, we will look at how you can make it easier on yourself when you begin the intermittent fasting eating pattern. It is daunting when you begin the intermittent fasting diet. Some people may experiment with the diet for three days and may not be hungry on the second day of their diet because they have done everything correctly. Instead of motivating yourself, you might tell yourself that you are going to fail because you are already hungry two hours after you broke your fast. There may be days when your hunger pangs were so strong that you could not make it through the fasting period. Some experts may tell you to switch to a high-fat diet, but it takes weeks for your body to adapt to such a diet and you cannot wait that long. Some people choose to back out even before they begin the diet because they are worried that they cannot see it through. What if there was a way to stay calm and confident when you start the diet?

Let us look at how you can do this. Instead of viewing the diet as another difficult path you owe to your health, perceive it as a self-experiment.

- Break the diet down into small and easy steps that will guarantee that you make it to the end of the diet

- Observe your body and analyze your findings

- Establish whether fasting is good for your body

In this instance, you are not committing to the diet, but are trying to learn more about it since people learn by doing. It does sound easier now.

Consult Your Doctor
As mentioned earlier, it is important to consult your doctor before you begin the diet. If you have a medical condition, you must create a plan that does not harm you further. If you feel sick or tired, you must stop the diet immediately.

Keep It Simple
When you are fasting, you must only consume plain water (with lemon juice or mint leaves if desired), black coffee or unsweetened tea. You must keep it this simple.

Keep It Easy
Eat the usual meals during the eating window. Experts suggest that you combine a low-carb and high-fat diet with intermittent fasting to reap benefits. You are only trying to finish the fast. When you decide the fast is good for you, you can look at combinations that work best for your body.

Create A Schedule
A schedule will keep your plan simple. You do not have to adhere to the time since your schedule may vary widely.

Days of The Week
It is easier to fast on weekdays than on weekends since the former are more structured and do not have any external factors affecting your fast. This may vary for you. You should look for days where you do not have the time to eat and fast only on those days.

It Is Okay to Slip Up
You must learn to forgive yourself. You can always pick up from where you dropped off and start the first day again. Try to do what is easiest for you to get back on track.

Identify Your Purpose
You must understand why it is important for you to follow the intermittent fasting diet.

Weight Maintenance or Weight Loss
Fasting helps to control the production of hormones like insulin, norepinephrine and HGH, which makes it easier for the body to burn stored fat and produce energy thereby helping you lose or maintain weight.

Avoid Medication and Relieve Symptoms
Fasting helps to reduce the risk of developing diabetes, heart diseases and inflammation.

Prevent Serious Diseases

Studies have shown that fasting protects the body from cancer and Alzheimer's. Some studies have also shown that fasting helps you live longer.

You must think about your reasons for starting the diet on days when you feel deprived.

Address Your Worries
What is it about intermittent fasting that makes you nervous and want to stop following the diet?

You Can Skip Breakfast
Breakfast is not the most important meal of the day. The reality is that you do not gain weight when you skip breakfast, and it does not help to kickstart your metabolism.

Avoid Snacks
Snacking, like breakfast, does not boost your metabolism and does not help you lose weight. Studies have shown that snacking leads to obesity and liver diseases.

Metabolism Does Not Slow Down
Fasting increases your metabolism and helps you retain muscle while you lose weight.

You should not be apprehensive about fasting because it is not hazardous to your health.

Learn to Be Patient

Again, with the patience theme, you need to be patient with sugar cravings. Cravings only tend to last an hour or so, and no matter how intense they come on, it's important to remember that they will subside! Give yourself an hour, distract yourself by going for a walk, or calling a friend and you may be surprised to see this craving dissipate.

Making Healthier Alternatives

When you're just starting out, it may be hard to kick these cravings overnight, and that's ok. Create healthy alternatives such as the recipes featured in the dessert section of this book. Choose rich foods like avocado to make an avocado pudding instead of indulging in ice cream. Swap in healthier alternative and soon your brain will be wired to crave the healthier version.

Eating Frequently

One of the biggest tricks to keeping sugar cravings at bay is to eat regularly. You want to eat small but frequent meals to keep your blood sugar levels stabilized. Your body will feel more satisfied, so you won't go into that starvation mode where you want to snack on all the wrong foods.

Whole Foods Are Always Better

Processed foods are full of artificial junk that can cause food cravings and blood sugar imbalances. Remove the processed foods from your diet and eat the real thing! You'll feel more satisfied, and your body will be much more nourished eating this way.

Steer Clear of All Artificial Sweeteners
Even though artificial sweeteners are often seen in fad diets, they aren't recognized by the body, and your body can't differentiate between artificial sugar and regular sugar. This can lead to sugar cravings. Remove these sweeteners altogether.

Supplements
Some supplements can help keep sugar cravings at bay. L-glutamine, omega 3's and green tea extract are a couple of commonly used supplements. Remember always to check with your doctor before starting any new supplements.

Get Sufficient Sleep
Often, sleep can be the reason you crave sweets. A lack of sleep can cause your hormones to be out of whack and can lead to cravings. Be sure to get quality uninterrupted sleep every single night to promote health and prevent cravings.

Exercise A Little
Exercise can help ward off sugar cravings as well. Activity raises your serotonin levels the same way a sugar binge does. By exercising regularly, you can keep your serotonin levels up naturally and fill that void without wanting to reach for junk.

Don't Eat Too Many Carbs

This is more of an obvious one, but one that happens quite frequently when you start eating a ketogenic diet. It occurs more if you don't take the proper steps in determining what your optimal net carb intake is. Once you know that number, it's harder to overeat carbohydrates. Remember to measure the number of ketones in your body, and as a rough estimate, the amount of carbs you can consume is between 20-50 grams per day.

Buy Seasonal Produce

If you are purchasing fruits and vegetables from a farmer or a farmer's market, then the product is bound to be seasonal. If you are picking these up from a supermarket, then you will never learn about seasonal produce. The only indication will be their price. The price of produce at the beginning of their respective season is higher since not much of it is available. Not only are out of season fruits and vegetables expensive, but they also lack in quality as well. Depending on where you reside, make sure that you learn a little about the local produce. Make sure that you are buying seasonal produce whenever possible.

Don't Overeat Protein

Although the ketogenic diet is based on low carb eating too much protein is not good either! When you eat more protein than your body requires, some of those extra amino acids will turn into glucose. This can throw your body out of ketosis, so don't go overdoing your post workout protein shakes! To be sure you aren't overeating in the protein department, try to stick with 0.7-0.9 grams of protein per pound of body weight and go for 0.9 grams of protein per pound if you are incredibly active.

Fats Are Your Friends

This diet is only valid if you eat the proper amount of fat! Don't be afraid of fat, especially healthy sources such as coconut, olive, and grass-fed butter. Your body needs this for energy, now that you are eliminating a vast majority of carbohydrate sources. Don't restrict fats or you will be in for some significant mood swings, you will always feel hungry, and your body will start to break down because it has nothing.

Don't Shop Without A List

Make sure that you have enough storage space for everything that you are planning on buying. Fresh food can be left on the shelf for a while, but most of the foods will need to be refrigerated. You can leave the eggs outside, but meat and fish need to be refrigerated. Always make a shopping list before you go shopping. It helps in buying only those ingredients that you need, instead of picking up random elements. Make a shopping list and stick to it. You can safely stay away from all sorts of junk if you do this. Take a couple of minutes and make a shopping list for yourself. There are mobile applications you can use.

Cheap Cuts of Meats

Following a new diet doesn't have to be an expensive affair. Expensive cuts of meats are certainly delicious, but please don't write off the cheaper cuts. Cuts like oxtail, pork shoulder or brisket are quite tasty when cooked properly, and they are certainly less expensive than regular cuts. Cook them in a pressure cooker or a slow cooker, and after a while, the meat will be falling off the bone. Offal and marrow bones are cheap too and they are full of nutrients. Offal is nutritious, but if you aren't keen on eating liver or any other offal you can always add it to other meats and vegetables while cooking. If you start shopping smartly, you can save a considerable sum of money.

Stay Away from Convenience Foods

Convenience foods are certainly an easy alternative. However, if you want to lose weight without burning a hole in your pocket, then it is better to cook your meals at home. If you manage to do your peal prep over the weekend and make a list of dishes you want to cook during the week, you will have your work cut out for you, and it will certainly make it easier to follow a diet.

If you start following these simple tips while starting your new diet, you will be able to increase your chances of success.

Chapter 16: Frequently Asked Questions

What is Intermittent Fasting?

As mentioned earlier, intermittent fasting is an eating pattern where you shift between periods of fasting and eating. This is not a diet that tells you what you should and should not eat but instead tells you how long you should avoid eating food. There are different types of patterns that you can choose from depending on what works best for you. These patterns are covered in Chapter Eleven. These patterns allow your body to spend more energy on healing and repair. This is not something that can happen if you are in the satiated state all the time.

Who is Intermittent Fasting For?

There are many benefits to following the intermittent fasting diet. These are covered in Chapter Eleven. If you are serious about improving your health and losing weight without making changes to your diet, you should consider the intermittent fasting eating pattern. Since you do not have to make too many changes to your diet, people prefer to follow the intermittent fasting eating pattern. If you want to burn the extra fat while maintaining your muscle, switch to this pattern. It is safe for everybody to follow and provides numerous benefits. The only thing you need to worry about is committing to the pattern, testing it and confirming whether this is something you can do regularly.

Why is It Effective?

Studies conducted in 2014 showed that intermittent fasting was effective since it had an impact on the adaptive cellular responses. This impact helped to reduce inflammation and oxidative damage, improve cellular production and optimize energy metabolism. This study was conducted in rodents, and it also showed that intermittent fasting helped to protect the animals from cancer, diabetes, neurodegeneration and heart diseases. Some studies conducted on human beings showed that intermittent fasting helped to reduce hypertension, obesity, rheumatoid arthritis and asthma.

The Journal of Nutritional Biochemistry published a study in the year 2005 that revealed that there are two reasons why intermittent fasting is effective – increased cellular stress resistance and reduced oxidative damage. This means that intermittent fasting will help your body deal well with stress and cope with fasting. As mentioned earlier, fasting triggers autophagy, which is the process where cells recycle or break cellular debris and dysfunctional protein. This is analogous to cleaning the house or taking the trash out. You should hope that this process happens in your body frequently. I hope this answer helped you understand how intermittent fasting works inside your body.

Why does Intermittent Fasting Burn Fat?

Chapter eleven covered the numerous benefits of intermittent fasting, and most of these benefits were centered on weight loss. Let us look at some of the other ways in which fasting helps to burn fat in the body:

- Increased levels of glucagon, which is a hormone that burns fat

- Increased number of uncoupling protein-3 mRNA, which is an important compound used to produce energy in a cell

- Increased epinephrine and norepinephrine levels that maximize the breakdown of fat

- Increased secretion of the sensitive lipase hormone

- Increased secretion of the growth hormone which helps to preserve a healthy metabolic rate and muscle mass

The idea behind fasting is that your body will begin to rely on the fat stores. Your body will experience this phenomenon when you exercise consistently. Your body will learn to attack the stored fat to provide the various organs with energy.

How Should I Fast to Lose Weight?

This is the same as what was mentioned earlier. The easiest way to perform intermittent fasting is too fast for twenty-four hours. Most studies have used the alternate day fasting method, where you do not eat on alternate days. You can, however, notice significant results when you fast only once every week. You can finish dinner and then start your fast. If you can make it all the way until dinner the following day, you are golden! You should remember that your body will begin to use the stored fat to produce fuel when you are in the fasted state. Therefore, you can burn more fat instead of sugar. This will become a freeing process.

What Should I Eat During the Eating Period?

One of the most important steps of switching into the intermittent fasting eating pattern is to identify how you can shift back into eating food after the fasting period. When you finish your fast, you should pretend that your fast did not happen. You should not compensate for the fasting period or reward yourself. You should wipe the fact that you were fasting a few minutes ago from your memory and eat the way you would normally eat during the day and ensure that you eat responsibly.

If you end the fast at dinnertime, you should eat dinner. If you choose to end your fast at 4 PM you cannot consume anything but a light snack since you can only consume dinner at 7 PM. You should never consume larger quantities of food than what you would normally eat at that time. You cannot end your fast in a few seconds. Therefore, the best thing to do is pretend that you were not fasting and eat the way you would normally eat at the time. Most people tend to crave healthier foods when they end their fast and choose a healthy snack or a smoothie instead of devouring a large tub of ice cream.

Is Intermittent Fasting Bad for Blood Sugar?

Not everybody has low blood sugar as we are led to believe. It is not a common issue with people. You should, however, check with your doctor if you are unsure. People can maintain their blood sugar levels if they are healthy regardless of whether they are fasting or performing intense exercises.

Studies have examined the effects of a twenty-four hour fast, and it was found that fasting did not lower the blood sugar levels. They found that the blood sugar levels did not dip below the 3.5mmol/Liter mark, which denoted that fasting did not lower the blood sugar levels.

Can I Exercise When I Follow the Intermittent Fasting Pattern?

Experts suggest that you perform different exercises even when you follow the intermittent fasting pattern. It is always good to include a variety of exercises, and both yoga and biking are good examples of exercises that will complement intermittent fasting. You should also go through some resistance training once or twice a week to prevent the loss of muscle. You will notice that your energy levels are lower when you exercise while following the intermittent fasting pattern. This is because your body will tap into the glycogen reserves to produce energy, which leads to fatigue. Exercising for short durations and at a high intensity in the fasted state is something you should explore. This will help you lose fat at a fast pace.

Plan Meals Around Workouts

Experts recommend that you perform cardio on an empty stomach, so it is a good idea to go for a jog early in the morning or book an early spin class if you are fasting. It is, however, important that you consume the right food the previous night.

When you know you are going to exercise the following day, you should always think about what you must eat the previous day. Your meals should depend on the intensity of your workout. For instance, if you decide to go for a run or a spin class the next day, you must replenish the glycogen stores with carbohydrates for dinner, which will help you have enough energy for the workout. When you perform cardio after a meal, your body will not have the power to digest, absorb and assimilate the nutrients since your muscles will demand blood flow. It is important to plan your meals to ensure that you do not damage or harm your body while performing the exercise.

The Workouts You Should Choose

If you do not feel lightheaded when you fast, you can perform any form of exercise without any worry. Many athletes find that they are stronger after they fast for an extended period (16 or 20-hour fast).

People are more focused and lucid after a fast. You will derive more benefits when you fast frequently.

If you follow a diet that is rich in carbohydrates for fuel, you must be careful when you perform intense exercises like CrossFit at the end of the fasting period since you may feel dizzy or nauseous. You feel this way when the glycogen stores have depleted, which often happens at the end of the fasting period. If you perform a less intensive exercise, your body will begin to burn stored fat to produce energy.

When to Stop

As mentioned earlier, it is important to listen to your body when it comes to exercise and too fast. One of the major risks is that you may develop low blood sugar if you do not provide your body with the right nutrition. For someone who is new to performing the exercise while following IF, it is recommended that you perform fewer intensive exercises to prevent the dip in blood sugar levels. If there is a sudden dip in blood sugar levels, there is a possibility that you may faint or feel lightheaded.

This does sound scary. It is for this reason that planning is extremely important. Regardless of how long the fasting period is, an important thing for people to consider is the first meal they will consume at the end of the fasting period and how that meal fits into their exercise schedule. It is important to eat complex carbohydrates, protein, healthy fat and fiber during the eating period. On the days when you exercise, you must include more complex carbohydrates, and consume protein and fat on rest days.

Regardless of how intense your exercise schedule is, listen to your body and plan your meals accordingly.

Why do I Get Hungry during my Fasting Period?

Since you are not eating any food and your stomach is empty, you may experience a small growl occasionally. Additionally, the hungry hormone ghrelin will respond to a lack of food in your stomach. It is because of this hormone that your body will begin to react differently, and it will make your brain think that you are starving. The hunger pangs will disappear once your body adjusts to the fasting period.

Why do I get a Headache when I am Fasting?

You should remember that not everybody gets a headache when they follow the intermittent fasting pattern. A lot of research has been conducted on headaches and Ramadan fasting. Women are more susceptible to headaches when compared to men during the fasting period. This is not because of dehydration and is mostly due to withdrawal symptoms. This is like the headaches that you will experience when you quit smoking or drinking abruptly.

If you experience headaches during the first few days of your fast, it is okay since your body is still getting used to the eating pattern. You can treat your headaches normally when you are not fasting. You must remember to get a lot of fresh air and drink lots of water during the fasting period.

Can I Drink?

You can drink, but you must ensure that there are no calories. This does not mean that you can drink diet soda since it is not okay. You should stick to herbal tea or water. Some people choose to drink black coffee, but I would not advise that. The caffeine will increase the levels of epinephrine in your body, which will aid in fat loss. It is, however, a better idea to not drink coffee since you are better off without it, especially because you will not be consuming much food.

You should focus on drinking herbal teas or water, and avoid milk, sweeteners and sugar. You should understand that this is a day of rest for your body, which means that you cannot consume calories of any kind.

Can I Take My Supplements When I Follow the Intermittent Fasting Pattern?

You can take your multivitamins, but it is always a good idea to give your body a little break. If you are taking multivitamins, probiotics or fish oil, give yourself a break for one day. This will also help to protect your body from developing any sensitivity to these supplements or ingredients.

How Often Should I Do Intermittent Fasting?

The answer to this question depends on the type of method you want to use, and if you choose to fast for twenty-four hours, you should stick to fasting once a week. Some people do choose to fast for forty-eight hours every week and have seen great results, but you should restrict yourself to those hours each week.

Why do I Catch a Cold when I Follow Intermittent Fasting?

When you fast, the blood begins to flow into your adipose tissue. Researchers believe that the blood flows into the adipose tissue to help move the fat into the muscles, so it can be burned as fuel. It is because of this that vasoconstriction will occur in your toes and fingertips to compensate for the blood flow, and it is for this reason that you catch a cold.

Will Intermittent Fasting Slow Down My Metabolism?

Despite all the benefits that we have covered, you might still wonder if the intermittent fasting eating pattern will slow your metabolism or bring it to a halt. You have probably been told to eat a small meal or snack every three hours to avoid putting on weight. This is thankfully untrue. The American Journal of Clinical Nutrition published a study in the year 2000 to understand the impact of fasting on resting energy expenditure. The resting energy expenditure is the amount of energy your body will need to carry out the basic functions when you are resting. The subjects were asked to fast for four days, and to most people's surprise, the subjects saw that their metabolism increased for the first three days. In another study, the subjects were asked to fast on alternate days for twenty-two days. The researchers concluded that there was no decrease in the subjects' metabolic rate. In addition to this, people who were on a resistance exercise program and a low-calorie diet did not see an increase in the metabolic rate, and these subjects were consuming at least 800 calories every day for twelve weeks.

In further studies, it was noticed that there was no change in the metabolic rate even if a person chose to skip breakfast. There was also no difference in the metabolic rate of people who chose to eat only two meals a day when compared to those who ate seven meals a day. In other words, food or lack of food does not have anything to do with your metabolic rate. Your metabolism is tied to your weight and muscle mass. If your lean mass goes up or down, your metabolism will also go up or down. I hope these studies showed you that short-term fasting does provide many benefits, and you do not have to worry about sabotaging your metabolism.

Is Intermittent Fasting Safe for Women?

This is a question that many women ask, and this is one of the most controversial questions surrounding intermittent fasting. People who advise women against intermittent fasting state that some studies show that intermittent fasting affects fertility. While this is true, what people do not realize is that all these studies only use the alternate day fasting method. In this method, women do not eat anything every other day. It is for this reason that their hormones act crazy, leading to fertility issues. A woman can fast for an entire day, and only do that once a week. This is safe, and there are no side effects that have been observed yet.

Some research has been conducted which talks about how short-term fasting affects a woman's menstrual cycle. These studies show that fasts that last for as long as seventy-two hours do not affect the menstrual cycle. Even longer fasts do not have an impact on the menstrual cycle of women who weigh a normal weight. Research shows that longer fasts will affect the menstrual cycle of women who are very lean. There is a lot of research, which shows that women of all shapes and sizes can switch to the intermittent fasting eating pattern if they are healthy. Women should only fast continuously for twenty-four hours, and not for longer than that.

If you are a woman and are unsure of whether you should follow the intermittent fasting diet, you can ease into this eating pattern by only fasting for eight or ten hours at a time. You can then increase the length of your fasting period as you see fit.

Should A Person Suffering from Hypothyroid Switch to Intermittent Fasting?

Every human being will be fine if his or her fast does not last longer than twenty-four hours. This is what you should know about fasting: the circadian rhythm is affected by light and food exposure, and some lifestyle practices will help to enhance the natural circadian rhythms. The following practices will help to enhance your circadian rhythm.

Light Entertainment
You should sleep in a dark room, and always get enough exposure to the sun during the day.

Daytime Feeding
You should always eat during daylight. This is to ensure that the light and food rhythms are synchronized.

Intermittent Fasting
You should always consume food during the daylight hours in your eight-hour eating window. A sixteen-hour fast will lead to lower insulin levels and lower blood sugar. The diurnal rhythm is affected if your body has an intense hormonal response to food.

People Say That Fasting Is Not Good If You Suffer from Adrenal Fatigue. Is It True?
This varies from person to person, but if you have full-blown adrenal fatigue, you should perhaps have a shorter fasting period, and have small quantities of food throughout the day to maintain the blood sugar levels.

Conclusion

The Mediterranean diet includes the consumption of liberal amounts of olive oil, fruits, vegetables, lean proteins (predominantly fish), dairy products, and a little bit of wine! This diet places emphasis on the consumption of whole and fresh foods and the reduction in the consumption of processed foods. A regular ketogenic diet recommends that at least 65-70% of your daily caloric needs must be from healthy fats, about 25% from proteins, and the rest from carbs. The keto diet eliminates the consumption of whole grains, starchy vegetables, and sugar in all forms.

A combination of these two diets is the Ketogenic Mediterranean diet. This diet encourages the consumption of healthy oils, green vegetables, lean meats, lots of fish, poultry, eggs, dairy products, and a moderate amount of red wine! Whole grains, starchy vegetables, and all sugars are excluded from the purview of this diet. It is essentially a high-fat and a low-carb diet.

This diet has plenty of health benefits to offer. Since this diet prescribes the consumption of foods that are rich in healthy fats, there will be an automatic reduction in your appetite and in the number of calories you consume. This in turn will help in weight loss. Also, there will be a reduction in the level of triglycerides in your body and your cholesterol levels will be under control. Not just that, this diet is helpful in controlling the levels of blood sugar and insulin in your body. It also helps in treating several brain disorders like Parkinson's, Alzheimer's, and even autism.

The Keto Mediterranean diet is quite a simple diet to follow and by making a few changes to your regular eating habits, you will be able to reap all the benefits that this diet has to offer.

As you come to the end of this book, we would like to thank you for using it as your source of information and guide for a Ketogenic Mediterranean diet. All the information in this book has been taken from reliable sources and will assist you in your transition towards a healthier diet. As you slowly implement the diet, you will see the difference it makes in your life. Remember to be patient and consistent in order to see real results. If you find this book helpful, please recommend it to your friends or family as well.

If you find this book helpful in anyway a review to support my endeavors is much appreciated.

Anti-Inflammatory Keto (30% More Effective)

Christine Moore

www.ingramcontent.com/pod-product-compliance
Lightning Source LLC
Chambersburg PA
CBHW020257030426
42336CB00010B/802